POCKET COMPANION TO ACCOMPANY

DAVIS'S DRUG GUIDE FOR NURSES

SEVENTH EDITION

WITH DRUG UPDATE 2001

JUDITH HOPFER DEGLIN, PharmD
Adjunct Clinical Instructor of Pharmacy Practice
University of Connecticut
School of Pharmacy
Storrs, Connecticut

APRIL HAZARD VALLERAND, PhD, RN
Wayne State University
College of Nursing
Detroit, Michigan

F. A. DAVIS COMPANY • Philadelphia

F. A. Davis Company
1915 Arch Street
Philadelphia, PA 19103
www.FADavis.com

Copyright ©2001 by F. A. Davis Company

All rights reserved. This book is protected by copyright. No part of it may be reproduced, stored in a retrieval system, or transmitted in any form or by any means, electronic, mechanical, photocopying, recording, or otherwise, without written permission from the publisher.

Printed in Canada

Last digit indicates print number 10 9 8 7 6 5 4 3 2
Publisher, Nursing: Robert Martone
Director of Production: Robert Butler
Managing Editor: Bette R. Haitsch
Developmental/SGML Editor: Elena Coler
Cover Designer: Louis J. Forgione

NOTE: As new scientific information becomes available through basic and clinical research, recommended treatments and drug therapies undergo changes. The authors and publisher have done everything possible to make this book accurate, up to date, and in accord with accepted standards at the time of publication. However, the reader is advised always to check product information (package inserts) for changes and new information regarding dose and contraindications before administering any drug. Caution is especially urged when using new or infrequently ordered drugs.

Authorization to photocopy items for internal or personal use, of specific clients, is granted by F. A. Davis Company for users registered with the Copyright Clearance Center (CCC) Transactional Reporting Service, provided that the fee of $.10 per copy is paid directly to CCC, 222 Rosewood Drive, Danvers, MA 01923. For those organizations that have been granted a photocopy license by CCC, a separate system of payment has been arranged. The fee code for users of the Transactional Reporting Service is 8036-0875/01 0 + $.10.

CONTENTS

*Because of space limitations, additional classes or drugs not represented in *Davis's Drug Guide for Nurses*, 7th edition, are provided in this *Pocket Companion*.

SECTION II: DRUGS NOT REPRESENTED IN DAVIS'S DRUG GUIDE FOR NURSES, 7TH EDITION*

{ } = Available in Canada only.

*Because of space limitations, additional classes or drugs not represented in *Davis's Drug Guide for Nurses*, 7th edition, are provided in this *Pocket Companion*.

SECTION I
Classifications

PHARMACOLOGIC PROFILE

General Use:

Drugs used during labor and delivery include tocolytic and oxytocic agents. Tocolytics suppress uterine muscle activity to prevent preterm labor. Oxytocics are used to stimulate uterine muscles to induce labor, control postpartum hemorrhage, terminate pregnancy, or to promote milk ejection in lactation.

General Action and Information:

Tocolytics include beta-sympathomimetics (ritodrine) and magnesium sulfate. Beta-sympathomimetics relax uterine smooth muscles by binding to beta$_2$-receptors. Oxytocics (prostaglandins, synthetic oxytocin, and methylergonovine) stimulate uterine smooth muscle contractions.

Contraindications:

Beta-sympathomimetics are contraindicated in women with a history of cardiac, renal, or hepatic disease and in migraines, hyperthyroidism, asthma, or hypertension. Oxytocin is contraindicated in hypersensitivity and in anticipated nonvaginal delivery. Ergot alkaloids are contraindicated in hypersensitivity, hepatic and renal impairment, hypertension, and cardiovascular disease. Ergots should not be used to induce labor.

Precautions:

Use cautiously in first and second stages of labor, cardiovascular disease, hypertension, and renal disease (oxytocin). Use cautiously in patients with diabetes (beta-sympathomimetics).

Interactions:

Oxytocin—Severe hypertension if given after vasopressors. Excessive hypotension if used concurrently with cyclopropane anesthesia. **Methylergonovine**—Excessive vasoconstriction may result when used with other vasopressors. **Beta-sympathomimetics (ritodrine)**—Additive adrenergic side effects with other sympathomimetics. Use with MAO inhibitors may result in hypertensive crisis.

NURSING IMPLICATIONS

Assessment

- Monitor frequency, duration, and force of contractions and uterine resting tone. Opioid analgesics may be administered for uterine pain.
- Monitor temperature, pulse, and blood pressure periodically throughout therapy for cervical ripening or termination of pregnancy.

Potential Nursing Diagnoses

- Knowledge deficit, related to medication regimen (Patient/Family teaching).

Implementation

- Administer RhoGAM into the deltoid muscle within 3 hr and up to 72 hr after delivery, miscarriage, abortion, or transfusion.
- Warm suppositories to room temperature just prior to use. Patient should remain supine for 10 min after vaginal suppository.
- Vaginal inserts are placed transversely in the posterior vaginal fornix immediately after removing from foil package. See monograph for dinoprostone for specific directions pertaining to administration.
- Endocervical gel is applied after determining degree of effacement. Do not administer above the level of the cervical os. Follow manufacturer's guidelines for administration.
- Wear gloves when handling unwrapped suppository and the gel to prevent absorption through the skin. Should skin contact, occur wash hands immediately.
- Administer intranasal oxytocin nasal spray by squeezing the bottle while the patient is in a sitting position.

Patient/Family Teaching

- Advise patient to administer oxytocin nasal spray 2–3 min prior to planned breast feeding. Patient should notify health care professional if milk drips form non-nursed breast or if uterine cramping occurs.
- Explain the purpose of cervical ripening and abortifacient medications with the need for vaginal exams. Advise patient to inform health care professional if contractions become prolonged.
- Provide emotional support.
- Instruct patient receiving abortifacients to notify health care professional immediately if fever and chills, foul-smelling discharge, lower abdominal pain, or increased bleeding occurs.

Evaluation

Effectiveness of therapy is demonstrated by: ■ Complete abortion ■ Cervical ripening and induction of labor ■ Effective letdown reflex ■ Prevention of preterm labor.

Agents Used during Pregnancy/Lactation Included in
Davis's Drug Guide for Nurses

abortifacients
carboprost 1172
dinoprostone 297

oxytocics
methylergonovine 631
oxytocin 740

miscellaneous
Rho D immune globulin 879

tocolytics
ritodrine, 1181

AGENTS USED IN THE MANAGEMENT OF IMPOTENCE*

PHARMACOLOGIC PROFILE

General Use:

Treatment of erectile dysfunction.

General Action and Information:

Sildenafil inhibits enzyme that inactivates cyclic guanosine monophosphate (cGMP). cGMP produces smooth muscle relaxation of the corpus cavernosum, which enhances blood flow and subsequent erection. Alprostadil is a prostaglandin that acts locally to relax trabecular smooth muscle and dilate cavernosal arteries.

Contraindications:

Hypersensitivity. Sildenafil should not be used concurrently with nitrates (nitroglycerin, isosorbide). Alprostadil should not be used concurrently with penile implants or in cases of structural or pathologic abnormalities of the penis.

Precautions:

Sildenafil should be used cautiously in patients with serious underlying cardiovascular disease, those already using antihypertensives or glipizide, and those with anatomic penile deformity. Use with caution in conditions associated with priapism and bleeding disorders or active peptic ulcer disease. Alprostadil should be used cautiously in patients with coagulation abnormalities.

Interactions:

Sildenafil blood levels may be increased by cimetidine, erythromycin, ketoconazole, and itraconazole. Increased risk of serious hypotension when sildenafil is used with nitrates. (Concurrent use is contraindicated.)

NURSING IMPLICATIONS

Assessment

- Determine erectile dysfunction prior to administration. Sildenafil has no effect in the absence of sexual stimulation.
- Exclude disorders of the vascular system and cavernous body damage prior to use of alprostadil, because the drug is ineffective with these disorders.

Potential Nursing Diagnoses

- Sexual dysfunction (Indications).
- Knowledge deficit, related to medication regimen (Patient/Family Teaching).

Implementation

- Sildenafil is administered PO. Dose is usually administered 1 hr prior to sexual activity. It may be administered 30 min to 4 hr before sexual activity.
- Alprostadil is injected into the dorsolateral aspect of the proximal third of the penis avoiding visible veins. Rotate injection sites from side to side. Dosage is determined in the prescriber's office.

Patient/Family Teaching

- Instruct patient taking sildenafil to take the medication 1 hr prior to sexual activity and not more than once a day.
- Advise patient that sildenafil has not been approved for use in women.

---

*Because of space limitations, additional classes or drugs not represented in *Davis's Drug Guide for Nurses*, 7th edition, are provided in this *Pocket Companion*.

- Caution patient not to take sildenafil concurrently with nitrates.
- Instruct patient using alprostadil that it is not to be used more that 3 times per week.
- Teach patient that priapism (prolonged erection of >60 min) is dangerous, and immediate medical assistance should be sought. Failure to treat priapism may result in permanent irreversible damage.
- Drugs to treat erectile dysfunction do not protect against transmission of sexually transmitted diseases. Counsel patient that protection against sexually transmitted disease and HIV infection should be considered.

Evaluation

Effectiveness of therapy can be demonstrated by: ■ Male erection sufficient to allow intercourse without evidence of adverse effects.

Agents Used in the Management of Impotence Included in *Davis's Drug Guide for Nurses*

alprostadil, 1168   sildenafil, 921

ANDROGENS/ANABOLIC STEROIDS*

PHARMACOLOGIC PROFILE

General Use:

Androgens (testosterone) are used to replace androgen deficiencies in hypogonadism. They are also used in endometriosis and for palliative treatment in metastatic breast cancer. Danazol, also an androgen, is used in the management of endometriosis, fibrocystic breast disease, and hereditary angioedema. Nandrolone (an anabolic steroid) is used to manage anemia associated with chronic renal failure.

General Action and Information:

Testosterone is necessary for the formation of the male sexual organs and for the development of primary and secondary male sex characteristics.

Contraindications:

Contraindicated in pregnancy and lactation; carcinoma of the prostate or male breast and hepatic disease; hypercalcemia; and coronary artery disease.

Precautions:

Use cautiously in elderly men who have an increased risk of prostatic hypertrophy and carcinoma and in patients with a history of liver or cardiac disease.

Interactions:

Increased sensitivity to oral anticoagulants, insulin, NSAIDS, and oral hypoglycemic agents. Use with adrenal corticosteroids may increase occurrence of edema. Danazol may increase cyclosporine levels. Nandrolone increases the risk of hepatotoxic reactions to drugs.

NURSING IMPLICATIONS

Assessment

- Monitor intake and output ratios, weigh patient twice weekly, and assess patient for edema. Report significant changes indicative of fluid retention.
- **Men:** Monitor for precocious puberty in boys (acne, darkening of skin, development of male secondary sex characteristics—increase in penis size, frequent erections, growth of body hair). Bone age determination should be measured every 6 mo to determine rate of bone maturation and effects on epiphyseal closure).
- Monitor for breast enlargement, persistent erections, and increased urge to urinate in men. Monitor for difficulty urinating in elderly men, because prostate enlargement may occur.
- **Women:** Assess for virilism (deepening of voice, unusual hair growth or loss, clitoral enlargement, acne, menstrual irregularity).
- In women with metastatic breast cancer, monitor for symptoms of hypercalcemia (nausea, vomiting, constipation, lethargy, loss of muscle tone, thirst, polyuria).
- **Danazol:** Assess for endometrial pain prior to and periodically throughout therapy.
- **Nandrolone:** Monitor responses for symptoms of anemia.

Potential Nursing Diagnoses

- Sexual dysfunction (Indications, Side Effects).
- Knowledge deficit, related to medication regimen (Patient/Family Teaching).

Implementation

- **General Info:** Range of motion exercises should be done with bedridden patients to prevent mobilization of calcium from the bone.
- Treatment of endometriosis or fibrocystic breast disease with danazol should be started during menstruation or preceded by a pregnancy test.
- **IM:** Administer deep IM into the gluteal muscle.
- **Transdermal:** Apply patch to clean, dry, hairless skin.

Patient/Family Teaching

- **General Info:** Advise the patient to report the following signs and symptoms promptly; in male patients, priapism (sustained and often painful erection) or gynecomastia; in female patients, virilism (which may be reversible if medication is stopped as soon as changes are noticed), hypercalcemia (nausea, vomiting, constipation, and weakness), edema (unexpected weight gain, swelling of the feet), hepatitis (yellowing of the skin or eyes and abdominal pain), or unusual bleeding or bruising.
- Explain rationale for prohibition of use for increasing athletic performance. Testosterone is neither safe nor effective, but this use has the potential risk of serious side effects.
- Advise diabetics to monitor blood for alterations in blood sugar concentrations.
- Emphasize the importance of regular follow-up physical exams, lab tests, and x-rays to monitor progress.
- Advise patient to use a nonhormonal form of contraception during therapy.
- Radiologic bone age determinations should be examined every 6 mo in prepubertal children to determine rate of bone maturation and effects on epiphyseal centers.
- **Transdermal:** Advise patient to notify health care professional if female sexual partner develops mild virilization.

---

*Because of space limitations, additional classes or drugs not represented in *Davis's Drug Guide for Nurses*, 7th edition, are provided in this *Pocket Companion*.

Evaluation

Effectiveness of therapy can be demonstrated by: ■ Resolution of the signs of androgen deficiency without side effects. Therapy is usually limited to 3–6 mo, followed by bone growth or maturation determinations. ■ Increase in activity tolerance. ■ Decrease in size and spread of breast malignancy in postmenopausal women. In antineoplastic therapy, response may require 3 mo of therapy; if signs of disease progression appear, therapy should be discontinued. ■ Decrease in symptoms of endometriosis. ■ Increased hemoglobin and red cell volume with decrease in symptoms of anemia.

Androgens/Anabolic Steroids Included in *Davis's Drug Guide for Nurses*

danazol 261   testosterone 966
nandrolone 687

ANESTHETICS/ANESTHETIC ADJUNCTS*

PHARMACOLOGIC PROFILE

General Use:

Anesthetics (general, local, regional) are used to induce anesthesia during surgery, childbirth, dental or diagnostic procedures, and other treatments. General anesthesia is administered parenterally or by inhalation to produce progressive and reversible stages of CNS depression. Local anesthetics (topical, injectable) produce anesthesia in small, localized areas. Regional anesthetics are used for larger areas (spinal, epidural). Anesthetic adjuncts are given preoperatively, intraoperatively, or postoperatively to aid in the anesthetic process. Anesthetic adjuncts (antianxiety and sedative/hypnotic agents, anticholinergic agents, narcotic analgesics, neuromuscular blocking agents) are used to enhance anesthetic agents.

General Action and Information:

Reversibly block transport of ions in neuronal membrane channels and thereby prevent initiation and conduction of normal nerve impulses.

Contraindications:

Hypersensitivity and cross-sensitivity may occur.

Precautions:

Use cautiously in patients with liver disease, cardiac disease, hyperthyroidism, respiratory depression, shock, or heart block. Use with caution in pregnancy or lactation (safety not established).

Interactions:

Additive CNS depression when administered with other CNS depressants. Additive cardiac depression and toxicity when administered with phenytoin, quinidine, procainamide, or propranolol.

NURSING IMPLICATIONS

Assessment

- Assess degree of numbness of affected part.
- Topical applications should have site assessed for open wounds prior to application. Apply only to intact skin.
- When using lidocaine/prilocaine, assess application site for anesthesia following removal of system and prior to procedure.
- In local epidural drugs, assess for systemic toxicity, orthostatic hypotension, and unwanted motor and sensory deficits.
- When using a systemic agent (propofol), assess respiratory status, pulse, blood pressure, and level of consciousness continuously throughout therapy and following administration.

Potential Nursing Diagnoses

- Pain, acute (Indications).
- Physical mobility, impaired (Adverse Reactions).
- Breathing patterns, ineffective (Adverse Reactions).
- Knowledge deficit, related to medication regimen (Patient/Family Teaching).

Implementation

- **Local Infiltration:** Epinephrine may be added to lidocaine to minimize systemic absorption and prolong local anesthesia.
- **Lidocaine/Prilocaine:** Apply dose in a thick layer at the site of the impending procedure and cover with an occlusive dressing at least 1 hr before the start of the procedure.
- **Epidural Medications:** Dose is titrated to patient response until anesthetic response is achieved.
- **Propofol:** Dose is titrated to patient response. Does not affect pain threshold, and adequate analgesia should always be used as an adjunct to surgical procedures. Shake well before IV administration, and use strict aseptic technique when administering.

Patient/Family Teaching

- **Local Block or Infiltrate:** Instruct patient to notify health care professional if any sensation of pain is felt.
- **Lidocaine/Prilocaine:** Explain the purpose of the of cream and occlusive dressing to patient and parents.
- **Epidural Medications:** Instruct patient to notify nurse if signs of systemic toxicity occur.
- **Propofol Use:** Inform patient that this medication will decrease recall of the procedure. Avoid use of alcohol or other CNS depressant agents for 24 hr following administration. Avoid driving or other activities requiring mental alertness for 24 hr after administration.

Evaluation

Effectiveness of therapy can be demonstrated by: ■ **Local Infiltration and Epidural Medication:** Complete blocking of pain sensation ■ **Lidocaine/Prilocaine:** Anesthesia in the area of application ■ **Propofol:** Induction maintenance of anesthesia; amnesia.

---

*Because of space limitations, additional classes or drugs not represented in *Davis's Drug Guide for Nurses*, 7th edition, are provided in this *Pocket Companion*.

Anesthetics/Anesthetic Adjuncts Included in *Davis's Drug Guide for Nurses*

Anesthetics (epidural)
bupivacaine 342
levobupivacaine 342
ropivacaine 342

Anesthetics (general)
ketamine 1177
propofol 844

Anesthetics (topical, mucosal)
lidocaine 577
lidocaine/prilocaine 579

ANGIOTENSIN-CONVERTING ENZYME (ACE) INHIBITORS

See Antihypertensive Agents, page C23.

ACE Inhibitors Included in *Davis's Drug Guide for Nurses*

benazepril 63
captopril 63
enalapril, enalaprilat 63
fosinopril 64
lisinopril 64

moexipril 64
perindopril 64
quinapril 64
ramipril 64
trandolapril 64

ANOREXIANTS*

PHARMACOLOGIC PROFILE

General Use:

Short-term management of exogenous obesity in conjunction with behavior modification, diet, and exercise.

General Action and Information:

Appetite suppression probably due to depression of CNS appetite control center (phentermine, phenylpropanolamine). Act as inhibitors of the reuptake of serotonin, norepinephrine, and dopamine and increase the satiety-producing effects of serotonin (sibutramine).

Contraindications:

Safety not established in pregnancy and lactation and in children under age 12.

Precautions:

Use cautiously in patients with cardiovascular disease (including hypertension), glaucoma, hyperthyroidism, diabetes mellitus, and prostatic hypertrophy.

Interactions:

Additive sympathomimetic effects with other adrenergic agents. Should not be used with MAO inhibitors. May increase the risk of hypertension with reserpine, tricyclic antidepressants, or ganglionic blocking agents.

NURSING IMPLICATIONS

Assessment

- Exclude hypertension and diabetes prior to instituting phentermine.
- Assess patient for weight loss, and adjust concurrent medications (antihypertensive agents, antidiabetic agents, lipid-lowering agents) as needed.
- Monitor nutritional intake periodically throughout therapy.
- **Sibutramine:** Monitor blood pressure and heart rate regularly during therapy. Increases in blood pressure or heart rate, especially during early therapy, may require decrease in dose or discontinuation of the drug.

Potential Nursing Diagnoses

- Body image disturbance (Indications).
- Nutrition, altered: more than body requirements (Indications).
- Knowledge deficit, related to medication regimen (Patient/Family Teaching).

Implementation

- Take once daily without regard to meals.
- **Phentermine:** Take once daily 30 min prior to breakfast or 10–14 hr before bedtime.

Patient/Family Teaching

- Instruct patient to take medication as directed and not to exceed recommended dose. Some medications may need to be discontinued gradually.
- **Sibutramine:** Caution patient to avoid using other CNS depresant or excessive amounts of alcohol.
- Advise patient to follow a reduced-calorie diet in conjunction with exercise, as recommended by their health care professional.
- **Phentermine and Phenylpropanolamine:** Warn patient to avoid large amounts of coffee, tea, or colas containing caffeine.

Evaluation

Effectiveness of therapy can be demonstrated by: ■ Slow, consistent weight loss when combined with reduced-calorie diet.

Anorexiants Included in *Davis's Drug Guide for Nurses*

phentermine 1179   sibutramine 919
phenylpropanolamine 788

ANTIANGINAL AGENTS

PHARMACOLOGIC PROFILE

General Use:

Nitrates are used to treat and prevent attacks of angina. Only nitrates (sublingual, lingual spray, or intravenous) may be used in the acute treatment of attacks of angina pectoris. Calcium chan-

---

*Because of space limitations, additional classes or drugs not represented in *Davis's Drug Guide for Nurses*, 7th edition, are provided in this *Pocket Companion*.

nel blockers and beta-adrenergic blockers are used prophylactically in long-term management of angina.

General Action and Information:

Several different groups of medications are used in the treatment of angina pectoris. The nitrates (isosorbide dinitrate, isosorbide mononitrate, and nitroglycerin) are available as a lingual spray, sublingual tablets, parenterals, transdermal systems, and sustained-release oral dosage forms. Nitrates dilate coronary arteries and cause systemic vasodilation (decreased preload). Calcium channel blockers dilate coronary arteries (some also slow heart rate). Beta-adrenergic blocking agents decrease myocardial oxygen consumption via a decrease in heart rate. Therapy may be combined if selection is designed to minimize side effects or adverse reactions.

Contraindications:

Hypersensitivity. Avoid use of beta blockers or calcium channel blockers in advanced heart block, cardiogenic shock, or untreated congestive heart failure.

Precautions:

Beta-adrenergic blockers should be used cautiously in patients with diabetes mellitus, pulmonary disease, or hypothyroidism.

Interactions:

Nitrates, calcium channel blockers, and beta-adrenergic blockers may cause hypotension with other antihypertensive agents or acute ingestion of alcohol. Verapamil, diltiazem, and beta-adrenergic blockers may have additive myocardial depressant effects when used with other agents that affect cardiac function. Verapamil has a number of other significant drug-drug interactions.

NURSING IMPLICATIONS

Assessment

- Assess location, duration, intensity, and precipitating factors of patient's anginal pain.
- Monitor blood pressure and pulse periodically throughout therapy.

Potential Nursing Diagnoses

- Pain (Indications).
- Tissue perfusion, altered (Indications).
- Knowledge deficit, related to medication regimen (Patient/Family Teaching).

Implementation

- Available in various dose forms. See specific drugs for information on administration.

Patient/Family Teaching

- Instruct patient on concurrent nitrate therapy and prophylactic antianginal agents to continue taking both medications as ordered and to use SL nitroglycerin as needed for anginal attacks.

- Advise patient to contact health care professional immediately if chest pain does not improve; worsens after therapy; is accompanied by diaphoresis or shortness of breath; or if severe, persistent headache occurs.
- Caution patient to make position changes slowly to minimize orthostatic hypotension.
- Advise patient to avoid concurrent use of alcohol with these medications.

Evaluation

Effectiveness of therapy can be demonstrated by: ■ Decrease in frequency and severity of anginal attacks ■ Increase in activity tolerance.

Antianginal Agents Included in *Davis's Drug Guide for Nurses*

beta-adrenergic blocking agents
atenolol 79
metoprolol 638
nadolol 678
propranolol 849

calcium channel blockers
amlodipine 41
bepridil 98

diltiazem 293
nicardipine 699
nifedipine 705
verapamil 1037

nitrates and nitrites
isosorbide dinitrate 539
isosorbide mononitrate 539
nitroglycerin 714

ANTI-ANXIETY AND SEDATIVE/HYPNOTIC AGENTS*

PHARMACOLOGIC PROFILE

General Use:

Antianxiety agents and sedatives are used to treat anxiety disorders and to provide sedation before procedures. Hypnotics are used to treat insomnia. Selected agents are useful as anticonvulsants (clorazepate, diazepam, phenobarbital), as skeletal muscle relaxants (diazepam), as adjuncts in the treatment of alcohol withdrawal syndrome (chlordiazepoxide, clorazepate, diazepam, oxazepam), and as general anesthetic adjuncts (droperidol) or amnestics (midazolam, dizepam).

General Action and Information:

Cause general CNS depression. May produce tolerance with chronic use and have potential for psychological or physical dependence. These agents have no analgesic properties.

Contraindications:

Hypersensitivity. Should not be used in comatose patients or in those with pre-existing CNS depression. Should not be used in patients with uncontrolled severe pain. Avoid use during pregnancy or lactation.

Precautions:

Use cautiously in patients with hepatic dysfunction, severe renal impairment, or severe underlying pulmonary disease. Use with caution in patients who may be suicidal or who may have had previous drug addictions. Hypnotic use should be short term. Geriatric patients may be more sensitive to CNS depressant effects (initial dosage reduction may be required).

---

*Because of space limitations, additional classes or drugs not represented in *Davis's Drug Guide for Nurses*, 7th edition, are provided in this *Pocket Companion*.

Interactions:

Additive CNS depression with alcohol, antihistamines, antidepressants, opioid analgesics, or phenothiazines. Barbiturates induce release of hepatic drug-metabolizing enzymes and can decrease the effectiveness of drugs metabolized by the liver. Should not be used with MAO inhibitors.

NURSING IMPLICATIONS

Assessment

- **General Info:** Monitor blood pressure, pulse, and respiratory status frequently throughout IV administration.
- Prolonged high-dose therapy may lead to psychological or physical dependence. Restrict the amount of drug available to patient, especially if patient is depressed, suicidal, or has a history of addiction.
- **Insomnia:** Assess sleep patterns before and periodically throughout therapy.
- **Anxiety:** Assess degree of anxiety and level of sedation (ataxia, dizziness, slurred speech) before and periodically throughout therapy.
- **Seizures:** Observe and record intensity, duration, and characteristics of seizure activity. Institute seizure precautions.
- **Muscle Spasms:** Assess muscle spasms, associated pain, and limitation of movement before and throughout therapy.
- **Alcohol Withdrawal:** Assess patient experiencing alcohol withdrawal for tremors, agitation, delirium, and hallucinations. Protect patient from injury.

Potential Nursing Diagnoses

- Sleep pattern disturbance (Indications).
- Injury, risk for (Side Effects).
- Knowledge deficit, related to medication regimen (Patient/Family Teaching).

Implementation

- Supervise ambulation and transfer of patients following administration of hypnotic doses. Remove cigarettes. Side rails should be raised and call bell within reach at all times. Keep bed in low position.

Patient/Family Teaching

- Discuss the importance of preparing environment for sleep (dark room, quiet, avoidance of nicotine and caffeine). If less effective after a few weeks, consult health care professional; do not increase dose. Gradual withdrawal may be required to prevent reactions following prolonged therapy.
- May cause daytime drowsiness. Caution patient to avoid driving or other activities requiring alertness until response to medication is known.
- Advise patient to avoid the use of alcohol and other CNS depressants concurrently with these medications.
- Advise patient to inform health care professional if pregnancy is planned or suspected.

Evaluation

Effectiveness of therapy can be demonstrated by: ■ Improvement in sleep patterns ■ Decrease in anxiety level ■ Control of seizures ■ Decrease in muscle spasm ■ Decrease in tremulousness ■ More rational ideation when used for alcohol withdrawal.

Anti-anxiety and Sedative/Hypnotic Agents Included in *Davis's Drug Guide for Nurses*

antihistamines
diphenhydramine 300
hydroxyzine 493
promethazine 893

barbiturates
pentobarbital 776
phenobarbital 784

benzodiazepines
alprazolam 23
chlordiazepoxide 188
diazepam 279

flurazepam 422
lorazepam 588
midazolam 645
oxazepam 735
temazepam, 735
triazolam 1016

miscellaneous
buspirone 131
doxepin 330
zaleplon 1064
zolpidem 1072

ANTIARRHYTHMIC AGENTS

PHARMACOLOGIC PROFILE

General Use:

Suppression of cardiac arrhythmias.

General Action and Information:

Correct cardiac arrhythmias by a variety of mechanisms, depending on the group used. The therapeutic goal is decreased symptomatology and increased hemodynamic performance. Choice of agent depends on etiology of arrhythmia and individual patient characteristics. Treatable causes of arrhythmias should be corrected before therapy is initiated (e.g., electrolyte disturbances). Major antiarrhythmics are generally classified by their effects on cardiac conduction tissue (see the following table). Adenosine, atropine, and digitalis glycosides (digitoxin, digoxin) are also used as antiarrhythmics.

MECHANISM OF ACTION OF MAJOR ANTIARRHYTHMIC DRUGS

GROUP	DRUGS	MECHANISM
I	moricizine	Shares properties of IA, IB, and IC agents
IA	disopyramide, procainamide, quinidine	Depress Na conductance, increase APD and ERP, decrease membrane responsiveness
IB	lidocaine, mexiletine, phenytoin, tocainide,	Increase K conductance, decrease APD and ERP
IC	flecainide, propafenone	Profound slowing of conduction, markedly depress phase O
II	acebutolol, esmolol, propranolol	Interfere with Na conductance, depress cell membrane, decrease automaticity, and increase ERP of the AV node, block excess sympathetic activity
III	amiodarone, bretylium, ibutilide, sotalol	Interfere with norepinephrine, increase APD and ERP
IV	diltiazem, verapamil	Increase AV nodal ERP, Ca channel blocker

APD = action-potential duration; Ca = calcium; ERP = effective refractory period; K = potassium; Na = sodium.

*Because of space limitations, additional classes or drugs not represented in *Davis's Drug Guide for Nurses*, 7th edition, are provided in this *Pocket Companion*.

Contraindications:

Differ greatly among various agents. See individual drugs.

Precautions:

Differ greatly among agents used. Appropriate dosage adjustments should be made in elderly patients and those with renal or hepatic impairment, depending on agent chosen. Correctable causes (electrolyte abnormalities, drug toxicity) should be evaluated. See individual drugs.

Interactions:

Differ greatly among agents used. See individual drugs.

NURSING IMPLICATIONS

Assessment

- Monitor ECG, pulse, and blood pressure continuously throughout IV administration and periodically throughout oral administration.

Potential Nursing Diagnoses

- Cardiac output, decreased (Indications).
- Knowledge deficit, related to medication regimen (Patient/Family Teaching).

Implementation

- Take apical pulse before administration of oral doses. Withhold dose and notify physician or other health care professional if heart rate is <50 bpm.
- Administer oral doses with a full glass of water. Most sustained-release preparations should be swallowed whole. Do not crush, break, or chew tablets or open capsules, unless specifically instructed.

Patient/Family Teaching

- Instruct patient to take oral doses around the clock, as directed, even if feeling better.
- Instruct patient or family member on how to take pulse. Advise patient to report changes in pulse rate or rhythm to health care professional.
- Caution patient to avoid taking OTC medications without consulting health care professional.
- Advise patient to carry identification describing disease process and medication regimen at all times.
- Emphasize the importance of follow-up exams to monitor progress.

Evaluation

Effectiveness of therapy can be demonstrated by: ■ Resolution of cardiac arrhythmias without detrimental side effects.

Antiarrhythmic Agents Included in *Davis's Drug Guide for Nurses*

group I	*group IA*
moricizine 665	disopyramide 306

procainamide 828
quinidine 868

group IB
lidocaine 577
mexiletine 644
phenytoin 790
tocainide 1002

group IC
flecainide 400
propafenone 841

group II
acebutolol 1
esmolol 363
metoprolol 638

propranolol 849

group III
amiodarone 35
bretylium 117
ibutilide 501
sotalol 935

group IV
diltiazem 293
verapamil 1037

miscellaneous
adenosine 11
atropine 81
digoxin 287

ANTICHOLINERGIC AGENTS

PHARMACOLOGIC PROFILE

General Use:

Atropine—Bradyarrhythmias. **Scopolamine**—Nausea and vomiting related to motion sickness and vertigo. **Propantheline and glycopyrrolate**—Decreasing gastric secretory activity and increasing esophageal sphincter tone. Atropine and scopolamine are also used as ophthalmic mydriatics.

General Action and Information:

Competitively inhibit the action of acetylcholine. In addition, atropine, glycopyrrolate, propantheline, and scopolamine are antimuscarinic in that they inhibit the action of acetylcholine at sites innervated by postganglionic cholinergic nerves.

Contraindications:

Hypersensitivity, narrow-angle glaucoma, severe hemorrhage, tachycardia (due to thyrotoxicosis or cardiac insufficiency), or myasthenia gravis.

Precautions:

Geriatric and pediatric patients are more susceptible to adverse effects. Use cautiously in patients with urinary tract pathology; those at risk for GI obstruction; and those with chronic renal, hepatic, pulmonary, or cardiac disease.

Interactions:

Additive anticholinergic effects (dry mouth, dry eyes, blurred vision, constipation) with other agents possessing anticholinergic activity, including antihistamines, antidepressants, quinidine, and disopyramide. May alter GI absorption of other drugs by inhibiting GI motility and increasing transit time. Antacids may decrease absorption of anticholinergics.

---

*Because of space limitations, additional classes or drugs not represented in *Davis's Drug Guide for Nurses*, 7th edition, are provided in this *Pocket Companion*.

NURSING IMPLICATIONS

Assessment

- Assess vital signs and ECG frequently during IV drug therapy. Report any significant changes in heart rate or blood pressure or increase in ventricular ectopy or angina promptly.
- Monitor intake and output ratios in elderly or surgical patients; may cause urinary retention.
- Assess patient regularly for abdominal distention and auscultate for bowel sounds. Constipation may become a problem. Increasing fluids and adding bulk to the diet may help alleviate constipation.

Potential Nursing Diagnoses

- Cardiac output, decreased (Indications).
- Oral mucous membrane, altered (Side Effects).
- Constipation (Side Effects).

Implementation

- **PO:** Administer oral doses of atropine, glycopyrrolate, propantheline, or scopolamine 30 min before meals.
- Scopolamine transdermal patch should be applied at least 4 hr before travel.

Patient/Family Teaching

- **General Info:** Instruct patient that frequent rinses, sugarless gum or candy, and good oral hygiene may help relieve dry mouth.
- May cause drowsiness. Caution patient to avoid driving or other activities requiring alertness until response to medication is known.
- **Ophth:** Advise patients that ophthalmic preparations may temporarily blur vision and impair ability to judge distances. Dark glasses may be needed to protect eyes from bright light.

Evaluation

Effectiveness of therapy can be demonstrated by: ■ Increase in heart rate ■ Decrease in nausea and vomiting related to motion sickness or vertigo ■ Dryness of mouth ■ Dilation of pupils ■ Decrease in GI motility ■ Resolution of signs and symptoms of Parkinson's disease.

Anticholinergic Agents Included in *Davis's Drug Guide for Nurses*

atropine 81	propantheline 843
glycopyrrolate 444	scopolamine 913

ANTICOAGULANTS

PHARMACOLOGIC PROFILE

General Use:

Prevention and treatment of thromboembolic disorders including deep vein thrombosis, pulmonary embolism, and atrial fibrillation with embolization.

General Action and Information:

Anticoagulants are used to prevent clot extension and formation. They do not dissolve clots. The two types of anticoagulants in common use are parenteral heparins and oral warfarin. Therapy is usually initiated with heparin because of its rapid onset of action, while maintenance therapy consists of warfarin. Warfarin takes several days to produce therapeutic anticoagulation. In serious or severe thromboembolic events, heparin therapy may be preceded by thrombolytic therapy (alteplase, anistreplase, streptokinase, or urokinase). Low doses of heparin, low-molecular-weight heparins, and heparin-like compounds (ardeparin, danaparoid, dalteparin, enoxaparin) are mostly used to prevent deep vein thrombosis after certain surgical procedures and in similar situations in which prolonged bedrest increases the risk of thromboembolism.

Contraindications:

Underlying coagulation disorders, ulcer disease, malignancy, recent surgery, or active bleeding.

Precautions:

Anticoagulation should be undertaken cautiously in any patient with a potential site for bleeding. Pregnant or lactating patients should not receive warfarin. Heparin does not cross the placenta. Heparin and heparin-like agents should be used cautiously in patients receiving epidural analgesia.

Interactions:

Warfarin is highly protein bound and may displace or be displaced by other highly protein-bound drugs. The resultant interactions depend on which drug is displaced. Bleeding may be potentiated by aspirin or large doses of penicillins or penicillin-like drugs, cefamandole, cefotetan, cefoperazone, plicamycin, valproic acid, or NSAIDs.

NURSING IMPLICATIONS

Assessment

- Assess patient taking anticoagulants for signs of bleeding and hemorrhage (bleeding gums; nosebleed; unusual bruising; tarry, black stools; hematuria; fall in hematocrit or blood pressure; guaiac-positive stools; urine; or nasogastric aspirate).
- Assess patient for evidence of additional or increased thrombosis. Symptoms will depend on area of involvement.
- **Lab Test Considerations:** Monitor activated partial thromboplastin time (aPTT) or international normalized ratio (INR) with full-dose heparin therapy, prothrombin time (PT) with warfarin therapy, and hematocrit and other clotting factors frequently during therapy.
- Monitor bleeding time throughout antiplatelet therapy. Prolonged bleeding time, which is time- and dose-dependent, is expected.
- **Toxicity and Overdose:** If overdose occurs or anticoagulation needs to be immediately reversed, the antidote for heparins is protamine sulfate; for warfarin, the antidote is vitamin K (phytonadione [AquaMEPHYTON]). Administration of whole blood or plasma may also be required in severe bleeding due to warfarin because of the delayed onset of vitamin K.

Potential Nursing Diagnoses

- Tissue perfusion, altered (Indications).

---

*Because of space limitations, additional classes or drugs not represented in *Davis's Drug Guide for Nurses*, 7th edition, are provided in this *Pocket Companion*.

- Injury, risk for (Side Effects).
- Knowledge deficit, related to medication regimen (Patient/Family Teaching).

Implementation

- Inform all personnel caring for patient of anticoagulant therapy. Venipunctures and injection sites require application of pressure to prevent bleeding or hematoma formation.
- Use an infusion pump with continuous infusions to ensure accurate dosage.

Patient/Family Teaching

- Caution patient to avoid activities leading to injury, to use a soft toothbrush and electric razor, and to report any symptoms of unusual bleeding or bruising to health care professional immediately.
- Instruct patient not to take OTC medications, especially those containing aspirin, NSAIDs, or alcohol, without advice of health care professional.
- Review foods high in vitamin K (see Appendix L) with patients on warfarin. Patient should have consistent limited intake of these foods, as vitamin K is the antidote for warfarin and greatly alternating intake of these foods will cause PT levels to fluctuate.
- Emphasize the importance of frequent lab tests to monitor coagulation factors.
- Instruct patient to carry identification describing medication regimen at all times and to inform all health care personnel caring for patient of anticoagulant therapy before lab tests, treatment, or surgery.

Evaluation

Clinical response can be evaluated by: ■ Prevention of undesired clotting and its sequelae without signs of hemorrhage ■ Prevention of stroke, myocardial infarction, and vascular death in patients at risk.

Anticoagulants Included in *Davis's Drug Guide for Nurses*

ardeparin 469	enoxaparin 469
dalteparin 469	heparin 465
danaparoid 469	warfarin 1057

ANTICONVULSANTS

PHARMACOLOGIC PROFILE

General Use:

See the following table.

General Action and Information:

Anticonvulsants include a variety of agents, all capable of depressing abnormal neuronal discharges in the CNS that may result in seizures. They may work by preventing the spread of seizure activity, depressing the motor cortex, raising seizure threshold, or altering levels of neurotransmitters, depending on the group. See individual drugs.

MAJOR ANTICONVULSANT CLASSES, DRUGS, AND MOST COMMON USES

CLASS	DRUGS	TYPE OF SEIZURE CONTROLLED
Barbiturates	phenobarbital	Tonic-clonic and partial seizures, prophylaxis of febrile seizures
Benzodiazepines	clonazepam	Absence seizures, akinetic seizures, myoclonic seizures
	clorazepate	Partial seizures
	diazepam (IV)	Status epilepticus, tonic-clonic seizures
	lorazepam (IV)	Status epilepticus
Hydantoins	fosphenytoin	Short-term parenteral management of seizures, treatment/prevention of seizures during neurosurgery
	phenytoin	Tonic-clonic and partial seizures with complex symptomatology
Succinimides	ethosuximide	Absence seizures
Miscellaneous	acetazolamide	Refractory seizures
	carbamazepine	Tonic-clonic seizures, complex partial seizures, mixed seizures
	gabapentin	Adjunctive treatment of partial seizures
	lamotrigine	Adjunctive treatment of partial seizures
	magnesium sulfate	Eclamptic seizures
	oxcarbazepine	Adjunctive therapy of partial seizures
	tiagabine	Adjunct treatment of partial seizures
	topiramate	Adjunctive therapy of partial-onset seizures
	valproates	Simple and complex partial seizures

Contraindications:

Previous hypersensitivity.

Precautions:

Use cautiously in patients with severe hepatic or renal disease; dosage adjustment may be required. Choose agents carefully in pregnant and lactating women. Fetal hydantoin syndrome may occur in offspring of patients who receive phenytoin during pregnancy.

Interactions:

Barbiturates stimulate the metabolism of other drugs that are metabolized by the liver, decreasing their effectiveness. Hydantoins are highly protein-bound and may displace or be displaced by other highly protein-bound drugs. Lamotrigine, tiagabine, and topiramate are capable of interacting with several other anticonvulsants. For more specific interactions, see individual drugs. Many drugs are capable of lowering seizure threshold and may decrease the effectiveness of anticonvulsants, including tricyclic antidepressants and phenothiazines.

NURSING IMPLICATIONS

Assessment

- Assess location, duration, and characteristics of seizure activity.
- **Toxicity and Overdose:** Monitor serum drug levels routinely throughout anticonvulsant therapy, especially when adding or discontinuing other agents.

Potential Nursing Diagnoses

- Injury, risk for (Indications, Side Effects).
- Knowledge deficit, related to medication regimen (Patient/Family Teaching).

*Because of space limitations, additional classes or drugs not represented in *Davis's Drug Guide for Nurses*, 7th edition, are provided in this *Pocket Companion*.

Implementation

- Administer anticonvulsants around the clock. Abrupt discontinuation may precipitate status epilepticus.
- Implement seizure precautions.

Patient/Family Teaching

- Instruct patient to take medication every day, exactly as directed.
- May cause drowsiness. Caution patient to avoid driving or other activities requiring alertness until response to medication is known. Do not resume driving until physician gives clearance based on control of seizures.
- Advise patient to avoid taking alcohol or other CNS depressants concurrently with these medications.
- Advise patient to carry identification describing disease process and medication regimen at all times.

Evaluation

Effectiveness of therapy can be demonstrated by: ■ Decrease or cessation of seizures without excessive sedation.

Anticonvulsants Included in *Davis's Drug Guide for Nurses*

barbiturates
phenobarbital 784

benzodiazepines
clonazepam 211
clorazepate 216
diazepam 279
lorazepam 588

hydantoins
phenyltoin/fosphenytoin 790

succinamide
ethosuximide 1175

valproates
divalproex sodium 1030
valproate sodium 1030
valproic acid 1030

miscellaneous
carbamazepine 149
gabapentin 433
lamotrigine 561
magnesium sulfate 595
oxcarbazepine 736
tiagabine 989
topiramate 1006

ANTIDEPRESSANTS

PHARMACOLOGIC PROFILE

General Use:

Used in the treatment of various forms of endogenous depression, often in conjunction with psychotherapy. Other uses include: ■ Treatment of anxiety (doxepin) ■ Enuresis (imipramine) ■ Chronic pain syndromes (amitriptyline, doxepin, imipramine, and nortriptyline) ■ Smoking cessation (bupropion) ■ Bulimia (fluoxetine) ■ Obsessive-compulsive disorder (fluoxetine, sertraline).

General Action and Information:

Antidepressant activity most likely due to preventing the reuptake of dopamine, norepinephrine, and serotonin by presynaptic neurons, resulting in accumulation of these neurotransmitters.

The two major classes of antidepressants are the tricyclic antidepressants and the SSRI(s). Most tricyclic agents possess significant anticholinergic and sedative properties, which explains many of their side effects (amitriptyline, doxepin, imipramine, nortriptyline). The SSRIs are more likely to cause insomnia (fluoxetine, fluvoxamine, paroxetine, sertraline).

Contraindications:

Hypersensitivity. Should not be used in narrow-angle glaucoma. Should not be used in pregnancy or lactation or immediately after myocardial infarction.

Precautions:

Use cautiously in older patients and those with pre-existing cardiovascular disease. Elderly men with prostatic enlargement may be more susceptible to urinary retention. Anticholinergic side effects (dry eyes, dry mouth, blurred vision, and constipation) may require dosage modification or drug discontinuation. Dosage requires slow titration; onset of therapeutic response may be 2–4 wk. May decrease seizure threshold, especially bupropion.

Interactions:

Tricyclic antidepressants—May cause hypertension, tachycardia, and convulsions when used with MAO inhibitors. May prevent therapeutic response to some antihypertensives. Additive CNS depression with other CNS depressants. Sympathomimetic activity may be enhanced when used with other sympathomimetics. Additive anticholinergic effects with other drugs possessing anticholinergic properties. **MAO inhibitors**—Hypertensive crisis may occur with concurrent use of MAO inhibitors and amphetamines, methyldopa, levodopa, dopamine, epinephrine, norepinephrine, desipramine, imipramine, guanethidine, reserpine, vasoconstrictors, or ingestion of tyramine-containing foods. Hypertension or hypotension, coma, convulsions, and death may occur with meperidine or other opioid analgesics and MAO inhibitors. Additive hypotension with antihypertensives or spinal anesthesia and MAO inhibitors. Additive hypoglycemia with insulin or oral hypoglycemic agents and MAO inhibitors. **Fluoxetine, fluvoxamine, bupropion, citalopram, paroxetine, sertraline**, or **venlafaxine** should not be used in combination with or within weeks of MAO inhibitors (see individual monographs). Risk of adverse reactions may be increased by **rizatriptan, naratriptan, sumatriptan**, or **zolmitriptan.**

NURSING IMPLICATIONS

Assessment

- Monitor mental status and affect. Assess for suicidal tendencies, especially during early therapy. Restrict amount of drug available to patient.
- **Toxicity and Overdose:** Concurrent ingestion of monamine oxidase inhibitors and tyramine-containing foods may lead to hypertensive crisis. Symptoms include chest pain, severe headache, nuchal rigidity, nausea and vomiting, photosensitivity, and enlarged pupils. Treatment includes IV phentolamine.

Potential Nursing Diagnoses

- Coping, ineffective individual (Indications).
- Injury, risk for (Side Effects).
- Knowledge deficit, related to medication regimen (Patient/Family Teaching).

---

*Because of space limitations, additional classes or drugs not represented in *Davis's Drug Guide for Nurses*, 7th edition, are provided in this *Pocket Companion*.

Implementation

■ Administer drugs that are sedating at bedtime to avoid excessive drowsiness during waking hours, and administer drugs that cause insomnia (fluoxetine, fluvoxamine, paroxetine, sertraline, MAO inhibitors) in the morning. Bupropion must be given in divided doses.

Patient/Family Teaching

■ Caution patient to avoid alcohol and other CNS depressants. Patients receiving MAO inhibitors should also avoid OTC drugs and foods or beverages containing tyramine (see Appendix L for foods) during and for at least 2 wk after therapy has been discontinued, as they may precipitate a hypertensive crisis. Health care professional should be contacted immediately if symptoms of hypertensive crisis develop.
■ Inform patient that dizziness or drowsiness may occur. Caution patient to avoid driving and other activities requiring alertness until response to the drug is known.
■ Caution patient to make position changes slowly to minimize orthostatic hypotension.
■ Advise patient to notify health care professional if dry mouth, urinary retention, or constipation occurs. Frequent rinses, good oral hygiene, and sugarless candy or gum may diminish dry mouth. An increase in fluid intake, fiber, and exercise may prevent constipation.
■ Advise patient to notify health care professional of medication regimen before treatment or surgery. MAO inhibitor therapy usually needs to be withdrawn at least 2 wk before use of anesthetic agents.
■ Emphasize the importance of participation in psychotherapy and follow-up exams to evaluate progress.

Evaluation

Effectiveness of therapy can be demonstrated by: ■ Resolution of depression ■ Decrease in anxiety ■ Control of bedwetting in children over 6 yr of age ■ Management of chronic neurogenic pain.

Antidepressants Included in *Davis's Drug Guide for Nurses*

tricyclic antidepressants
amitriptyline 39
doxepin 330
imipramine 509
nortriptyline 719

selective serotonin reuptake inhibitors
citalopram 202
fluoxetine 417
fluvoxamine 426
paroxetine 752
sertraline 916

monoamine oxidase (MAO) inhibitors
phenelzine 661
tranylcypromine 661

miscellaneous
bupropion 129
mirtazapine 654
nefazodone 690
trazodone 1015
venlafaxine 1035

ANTIDIABETIC AGENTS

PHARMACOLOGIC PROFILE

General Use:

Insulin is used in the management of insulin-dependent diabetes mellitus (IDDM, type 1). It may also be used in non–insulin-dependent diabetes mellitus (NIDDM, type 2) when diet and/or oral hypoglycemic therapy fails to adequately control blood sugar. The choice of insulin preparation (rapid-acting, intermediate-acting, long-acting) and source (beef, beef/pork, pork, semisynthetic, human recombinant DNA) depend on the degree of control desired, daily blood sugar fluctuations, and history of previous reactions. Oral hypoglycemics can be used only in NIDDM, type 2. Oral agents are used when diet therapy alone fails to control blood sugar or symptoms or when patients are not amenable to using insulin. Some oral agents may be used with insulin.

General Action and Information:

Insulin, a hormone produced by the pancreas, lowers blood glucose by increasing transport of glucose into cells and promotes the conversion of glucose to glycogen. It also promotes the conversion of amino acids to proteins in muscle, stimulates triglyceride formation, and inhibits the release of free fatty acids. Sulfonylureas, repaglinide, and metformin lower blood sugar by stimulating endogenous insulin secretion by beta cells of the pancreas and by increasing sensitivity to insulin at intracellular receptor sites. Intact pancreatic function is required. Miglitol delays digestion of ingested carbohydrates, thus lowering blood sugar, especially after meals. It may be combined with sulfonylureas.

Contraindications:

Insulin—Hypoglycemia. **Oral hypoglycemic agents**—Hypersensitivity (cross-sensitivity with other sulfonylureas and sulfonamides may exist). Hypoglycemia. IDDM, type 1. Avoid use in patients with severe kidney, liver, thyroid, and other endocrine dysfunction. Should not be used in pregnancy or lactation.

Precautions:

Insulin—Infection, stress, or changes in diet may alter requirements. **Oral hypoglycemic agents**—Use cautiously in geriatric patients. Dosage reduction may be necessary. Infection, stress, or changes in diet may alter requirements. Use with sulfonylureas with caution in patients with a history of cardiovascular disease. Metformin may cause lactic acidosis.

Interactions:

Insulin—Additive hypoglycemic effects with oral hypoglycemic agents. **Oral hypoglycemic agents**—Ingestion of alcohol may result in disulfiram-like reaction with some agents. Alcohol, corticosteroids, rifampin, glucagon, and thiazide diuretics may decrease effectiveness. Anabolic steroids, chloramphenicol, clofibrate, MAO inhibitors, most NSAIDs, salicylates, sulfonamides, and warfarin may increase hypoglycemic effect. Beta-adrenergic blocking agents may produce hypoglycemia and mask signs and symptoms.

---

*Because of space limitations, additional classes or drugs not represented in *Davis's Drug Guide for Nurses*, 7th edition, are provided in this *Pocket Companion*.

NURSING IMPLICATIONS

Assessment

- Observe patient for signs and symptoms of hypoglycemic reactions.
- Miglitol and pioglitazone do not cause hypoglycemia when taken alone but may increase the hypoglycemic effect of other hypoglycemic agents.
- Patients who have been well controlled on metformin but develop illness or laboratory abnormalities should be assessed for ketoacidosis or lactic acidosis. Assess serum electrolytes, ketones, glucose, and, if indicated, blood pH, lactate, pyruvate, and metformin levels. If either form of acidosis is present, discontinue metformin immediately and treat acidosis.
- **Lab Test Considerations:** Serum glucose and glycosylated hemoglobin should be monitored periodically throughout therapy to evaluate effectiveness of treatment.

Potential Nursing Diagnoses

- Nutrition, altered: more than body requirements (Indications).
- Knowledge deficit: related to medication regimen (Patient/Family Teaching).
- Noncompliance (Patient/Family Teaching).

Implementation

- **General Info:** Patients stabilized on a diabetic regimen who are exposed to stress, fever, trauma, infection, or surgery may require sliding scale insulin. Withhold metformin and reinstitute after resolution of acute episode.
- Patients switching from daily insulin dose may require gradual conversion to oral hypoglycemics.
- **Insulin:** Available in different types and strengths and from different species. Check type, species' source, dose, and expiration date with another licensed nurse. Do not interchange insulins without physician's order. Use only insulin syringes to draw up dose. Use only U100 syringes to draw up insulin lispro dose.

Patient/Family Teaching

- **General Info:** Explain to patient that medication controls hyperglycemia but does not cure diabetes. Therapy is long-term.
- Review signs of hypoglycemia and hyperglycemia with patient. If hypoglycemia occurs, advise patient to take a glass of orange juice or 2–3 tsp of sugar, honey, or corn syrup dissolved in water (glucose, not table sugar, if taking miglitol), and notify health care professional.
- Encourage patient to follow prescribed diet, medication, and exercise regimen to prevent hypoglycemic or hyperglycemic episodes.
- Instruct patient in proper testing of serum glucose and ketones.
- Advise patient to notify health care professional if nausea, vomiting, or fever develops; if unable to eat usual diet; or if blood sugar levels are not controlled.
- Advise patient to carry sugar or a form of glucose and identification describing medication regimen at all times.
- Insulin is the recommended method of controlling blood sugar during pregnancy. Counsel female patients to use a form of contraception other than oral contraceptives and to notify health care professional promptly if pregnancy is planned or suspected.
- **Insulin:** Instruct patient on proper technique for administration; include type of insulin, equipment (syringe and cartridge pens), storage, and syringe disposal. Discuss the importance of not changing brands of insulin or syringes, selection and rotation of injection sites, and compliance with therapeutic regimen.

- **Sulfonylureas:** Advise patient that concurrent use of alcohol may cause a disulfiram-like reaction (abdominal cramps, nausea, flushing, headache, and hypoglycemia).
- **Metformin:** Explain to patient the risk of lactic acidosis and the potential need for discontinuation of metformin therapy if a severe infection, dehydration, or severe or continuing diarrhea occurs or if medical tests or surgery is required.

Evaluation

Effectiveness of therapy can be demonstrated by: ■ Control of blood glucose levels without the appearance of hypoglycemic or hyperglycemic episodes.

Antidiabetic Agents Included in *Davis's Drug Guide for Nurses*

alpha-glucosidase inhibitor
miglitol 649

biguanide
metformin 619

insulin mixture
NPH/regular insulin mixture 520

intermediate-acting insulin
insulin, NPH (isophane insulin suspension) 520
insulin zinc suspension (lente insulin) 520

long-acting insulin
insulin zinc suspension, extended (ultralenle insulin) 520

rapid-acting insulin
insulin, lispro, rDNA origin 520
regular insulin (insulin injection, crystalline zinc insulin) 520

sulfonylureas
glimepiride 495
glipizide 495
glyburide 495

miscellaneous
pioglitazone 801
repaglinide 877
rosiglitazone P–105

ANTIDIARRHEAL AGENTS

PHARMACOLOGIC PROFILE

General Use:

For the control and symptomatic relief of acute and chronic nonspecific diarrhea.

General Action and Information:

Diphenoxylate/atropine, difenoxin/atropine, and loperamide slow intestinal motility and propulsion. Kaolin/pectin and bismuth subsalicylate affect fluid content of the stool. Polycarbophil acts as an antidiarrheal by taking on water within the bowel lumen to create a formed stool. Octreotide is used specifically for diarrhea associated with GI endocrine tumors.

Contraindications:

Previous hypersensitivity. Severe abdominal pain of unknown cause, especially when associated with fever.

---

*Because of space limitations, additional classes or drugs not represented in *Davis's Drug Guide for Nurses*, 7th edition, are provided in this *Pocket Companion*.

Precautions:

Use cautiously in patients with severe liver disease or inflammatory bowel disease. Safety in pregnancy and lactation not established (diphenoxylate/atropine and loperamide). Octreotide may aggravate gallbladder disease.

Interactions:

Kaolin/pectin may decrease absorption of digoxin. Polycarbophil decreases the absorption of tetracycline. Octreotide may alter the response to insulin or oral hypoglycemic agents.

NURSING IMPLICATIONS

Assessment

- Assess the frequency and consistency of stools and bowel sounds before and throughout therapy.
- Assess patient's fluid and electrolyte status and skin turgor for dehydration.

Potential Nursing Diagnoses

- Diarrhea (Indications).
- Constipation (Side Effects).
- Knowledge deficit, related to medication regimen (Patient/Family Teaching).

Implementation

- Shake liquid preparations before administration.

Patient/Family Teaching

- Instruct patient to notify health care professional if diarrhea persists; or if fever, abdominal pain, or palpitations occur.

Evaluation

Effectiveness of therapy can be demonstrated by: ∎ Decrease in diarrhea.

Antidiarrheal Agents Included in *Davis's Drug Guide for Nurses*

attapulgite 1171
bismuth subsalicylate 110
difenoxin/atropine 303
diphenoxylate/atropine 303

kaolin/pectin 547
loperamide 585
octreotide 723
polycarbophil 811

ANTIDOTES

PHARMACOLOGIC PROFILE

General Use:

See the following table.

General Action and Information:

Antidotes are used in accidental and intentional overdoses of medications or toxic substances. The goal of antidotal therapy is to decrease systemic complications of the overdosage while supporting vital functions. Obtaining a precise history will determine aggressiveness of therapy, choice, and dose of agent. Some antidotes are designed to aid removal of the offending agent before systemic absorption occurs or to speed elimination (activated charcoal). Other agents are more specific and require more detailed history as to type and amount of agent ingested.

POISONS AND SPECIFIC ANTIDOTES

POISON	ANTIDOTE
acetaminophen	acetylcysteine
anticholinesterases	atropine, pralidoxime
benzodiazepines	flumazenil
cyclophosphamide	mesna
digoxin, digitoxin	digoxin immune Fab
doxorubicin	dexrazoxane
fluorouracil	leucovorin calcium
heparin	protamine sulfate
iron	deferoxamine
lead	succimer
methotrexate	leucovorin calcium
opiod analgesics, heroin	naloxone
warfarin	phytonadione (vitamin K)

Contraindications:

See individual drugs.

Precautions:

See individual drugs.

Interactions:

See individual drugs.

NURSING IMPLICATIONS

Assessment

- Inquire as to the type of drug or poison and time of ingestion.
- Consult reference, poison control center, or physician for symptoms of toxicity of ingested agent(s) and antidote. Monitor vital signs, affected systems, and serum levels closely.
- Monitor for suicidal ideation; institute suicide precautions as necessary.

Potential Nursing Diagnoses

- Coping, ineffective individual (Indications).
- Injury, risk for: poisoning (Patient/Family Teaching).
- Knowledge deficit, related to medication regimen (Patient/Family Teaching).

---

*Because of space limitations, additional classes or drugs not represented in *Davis's Drug Guide for Nurses*, 7th edition, are provided in this *Pocket Companion*.

Implementation

- May be used in conjunction with induction of emesis or gastric aspiration and lavage, cathartics, agents to modify urine pH, and supportive measures for respiratory and cardiac effects of overdose or poisoning.

Patient/Family Teaching

- When counseling about poisoning in the home, discuss methods of prevention and the need to confer with poison control center, physician, or emergency department prior to administering syrup of ipecac and the need to bring ingested substance to the hospital for identification. Reinforce need to keep all medications and hazardous substances out of the reach of children.

Evaluation

Effectiveness of therapy is demonstrated by: ■ Prevention or resolution of toxic side effects of ingested agent.

Antidotes Included in *Davis's Drug Guide for Nurses*

acetylcysteine 5
amyl nitrate 1170
deferoxamine 268
dexrazoxane 274
digoxin immune Fab 291
dimercaprol 1174
edetate calcium disodium 1175
flumazenil 406

leucovorin calcium 567
mesna 616
naloxone 685
pralidoxime 1180
protamine sulfate 854
sodium nitrate 1181
sodium thiosulfate 1181
succimer 939

ANTIEMETIC AGENTS

PHARMACOLOGIC PROFILE

General Use:

Phenothiazines, dolasetron, granisetron, metoclopramide, trimethobenzamide, and ondansetron are used to manage nausea and vomiting of many causes, including surgery, anesthesia, and antineoplastic and radiation therapy. Dimenhydrinate, scopolamine, and meclizine are used almost exclusively to prevent motion sickness.

General Action and Information:

Phenothiazines act on the chemoreceptor trigger zone to inhibit nausea and vomiting. Dimenhydrinate, scopolamine, and meclizine act as antiemetics mainly by diminishing motion sickness. Metoclopramide decreases nausea and vomiting by its effects on gastric emptying. Dolasetron, granisetron, and ondansetron block the effects of serotonin.

Contraindications:

Previous hypersensitivity.

Precautions:

Use phenothiazines cautiously in children who may have viral illnesses. Choose agents carefully in pregnant patients (no agents are approved for safe use).

Interactions:

Additive CNS depression with other CNS depressants including antidepressants, antihistamines, opioid analgesics, and sedative/hypnotics. Phenothiazines may produce hypotension when used with antihypertensives, nitrates, or acute ingestion of alcohol.

NURSING IMPLICATIONS

Assessment

- Assess nausea, vomiting, bowel sounds, and abdominal pain before and following administration.
- Monitor hydration status and intake and output. Patients with severe nausea and vomiting may require IV fluids in addition to antiemetics.

Potential Nursing Diagnoses

- Fluid volume deficit (Indications).
- Nutrition, altered: less than body requirements (Indications).
- Injury, risk for (Side Effects).

Implementation

- For prophylactic administration, follow directions for specific drugs so that peak effect corresponds to time of anticipated nausea.
- Phenothiazines should be discontinued 48 hr before and not resumed for 24 hr following myelography, as they lower seizure threshold.

Patient/Family Teaching

- Advise patient and family to use general measures to decrease nausea (begin with sips of liquids and small, nongreasy meals; provide oral hygiene; and remove noxious stimuli from environment).
- May cause drowsiness. Advise patient to call for assistance when ambulating and to avoid driving or other activities requiring alertness until response to medication is known.
- Advise patient to make position changes slowly to minimize orthostatic hypotension.

Evaluation

Effectiveness of therapy can be demonstrated by: ■ Prevention of, or decrease in, nausea and vomiting.

Antiemetic Agents Included in *Davis's Drug Guide for Nurses*

anticholinergic
scopolamine 913

antihistamines
dimenhydrinate 296
meclizine 604

---

*Because of space limitations, additional classes or drugs not represented in *Davis's Drug Guide for Nurses*, 7th edition, are provided in this *Pocket Companion*.

phenothiazines
chlorpromazine 191
prochlorperazine 833
promethazine 839
thiethylperazine 976
trifluoperazine 1018

serotonin (5-HT₃) antagonists

serotonin (5-HT$_3$) antagonists
dolasetron 323
granisetron 448
ondansetron 728

miscellaneous
benzquinamide 1171
cyclizine 1173
metoclopramide 634
trimethobenzamide 1022

ANTIFUNGAL AGENTS

PHARMACOLOGIC PROFILE

General Use:

Treatment of fungal infections. Infections of skin or mucous membranes may be treated with topical or vaginal preparations. Deep-seated or systemic infections require oral or parenteral therapy. New parenteral formulations of amphotericin employ lipid encapsulation technology designed to decrease toxicity.

General Action and Information:

Kill (fungicidal) or stop growth of (fungistatic) susceptible fungi by affecting the permeability of the fungal cell membrane or protein synthesis within the fungal cell itself.

Contraindications:

Previous hypersensitivity.

Precautions:

Because most systemic antifungals may have adverse effects on bone marrow function, use cautiously in patients with depressed bone marrow reserve. Amphotericin B commonly causes renal impairment. Fluconazole requires dosage adjustment in the presence of renal impairment. Adverse reactions to fluconazole may be more severe in HIV-positive patients.

Interactions:

Differ greatly among various agents. See individual drugs.

NURSING IMPLICATIONS

Assessment

■ Assess patient for signs of infection and assess involved areas of skin and mucous membranes before and throughout therapy. Increased skin irritation may indicate need to discontinue medication.

Potential Nursing Diagnoses

■ Infection, risk for (Indications).
■ Skin integrity, impaired (Indications).

- Knowledge deficit, related to medication regimen (Patient/Family Teaching).

Implementation

- **General Info:** Available in various dosage forms. Refer to specific drugs for directions for administration.
- **Topical:** Consult physician or other health care professional for cleansing technique before applying medication. Wear gloves during application. Do not use occlusive dressings unless specified by physician or other health care professional.

Patient/Family Teaching

- Instruct patient on proper use of medication form.
- Instruct patient to continue medication as directed for full course of therapy, even if feeling better.
- Advise patient to report increased skin irritation or lack of therapeutic response to health care professional.

Evaluation

Effectiveness of therapy can be demonstrated by: ■ Resolution of signs and symptoms of infection. Length of time for complete resolution depends on organism and site of infection. Deep-seated fungal infections may require prolonged therapy (weeks–months). Recurrent fungal infections may be a sign of serious systemic illness.

Antifungal Agents Included in *Davis's Drug Guide for Nurses*

ophthalmic antifungal
natamycin 1158

systemic antifungals
amphotericin B cholesteryl sulfate 48
amphotericin B deoxycholate 48
amphotericin B lipid complex 48
amphotericin B liposome 48
dapsone 1173
fluconazole 402
griseofulvin 450
itraconazole 543
ketoconazole 548

topical antifungals
amphotericin B deoxycholate 48
butenafine 70
ciclopirox 70
clotrimazole 70

econazole 70
haloprogin 70
ketoconazole 548
miconazole 70
naftifine 70
nystatin 721
oxiconazole 70
sulconazole 70
terbinafine 70
tolnaftate 70

vaginal antifungals
butoconazole 73
clotrimazole 73
miconazole 73
nystatin 721
terconazole 73
tioconazole 73

---

*Because of space limitations, additional classes or drugs not represented in *Davis's Drug Guide for Nurses*, 7th edition, are provided in this *Pocket Companion*.

ANTIHISTAMINES

PHARMACOLOGIC PROFILE

General Use:

Relief of symptoms associated with allergies, including rhinitis, urticaria, and angioedema, and as adjunctive therapy in anaphylactic reactions. Some antihistamines are used to treat motion sickness (dimenhydrinate and meclizine), insomnia (diphenhydramine), Parkinson-like reactions (diphenhydramine), and other nonallergic conditions.

General Action and Information:

Antihistamines block the effects of histamine at the H_1 receptor. They do not block histamine release, antibody production, or antigen-antibody reactions. Most antihistamines have anticholinergic properties and may cause constipation, dry eyes, dry mouth, and blurred vision. In addition, many antihistamines cause sedation. Some phenothiazines have strong antihistaminic properties (hydroxyzine and promethazine).

Contraindications:

Hypersensitivity and narrow-angle glaucoma. Should not be used in premature or newborn infants.

Precautions:

Elderly patients may be more susceptible to adverse anticholinergic effects of antihistamines. Use cautiously in patients with pyloric obstruction, prostatic hypertrophy, hyperthyroidism, cardiovascular disease, or severe liver disease. Use cautiously in pregnancy and lactation.

Interactions:

Additive sedation when used with other CNS depressants, including alcohol, antidepressants, opioid analgesics, and sedative/hypnotics. MAO inhibitors prolong and intensify the anticholinergic properties of antihistamines.

NURSING IMPLICATIONS

Assessment

- **General Info:** Assess allergy symptoms (rhinitis, conjunctivitis, hives) before and periodically throughout therapy.
- Monitor pulse and blood pressure before initiating and throughout IV therapy.
- Assess lung sounds and character of bronchial secretions. Maintain fluid intake of 1500–2000 ml/day to decrease viscosity of secretions.
- **Nausea and Vomiting:** Assess degree of nausea and frequency and amount of emesis when administering for nausea and vomiting.
- **Anxiety:** Assess mental status, mood, and behavior when administering for anxiety.
- **Pruritus:** Observe the character, location, and size of affected area when administering for pruritic skin conditions.

Potential Nursing Diagnoses

- Airway clearance, ineffective (Indications).

- Injury, risk for (Adverse Reactions).
- Knowledge deficit, related to medication regimen (Patient/Family Teaching).

Implementation

- When used for prophylaxis of motion sickness, administer at least 30 min and preferably 1–2 hr before exposure to conditions that may precipitate motion sickness.
- When administering concurrently with opioid analgesics (hydroxyzine, promethazine), supervise ambulation closely to prevent injury secondary to increased sedation.

Patient/Family Teaching

- Inform patient that drowsiness may occur. Avoid driving or other activities requiring alertness until response to drug is known.
- Caution patient to avoid using concurrent alcohol or CNS depressants.
- Advise patient that good oral hygiene, frequent rinsing of mouth with water, and sugarless gum or candy may help relieve dryness of mouth.
- Instruct patient to contact health care professional if symptoms persist.

Evaluation

Effectiveness of therapy can be demonstrated by: ■ Decrease in allergic symptoms ■ Prevention or decreased serverity of nausea and vomiting ■ Decrease in anxiety ■ Relief of pruritus ■ Sedation when used as a sedative/hypnotic.

Antihistamines Included in *Davis's Drug Guide for Nurses*

azatadine 84	diphenhydramine 300
brompheniramine 118	fexofenadine P–95
cetirizine 183	hydroxyzine 493
chlorpheniramine 190	loratadine 587
cyproheptadine 254	meclizine 604
dimenhydrinate 296	promethazine 839

ANTIHYPERTENSIVE AGENTS

PHARMACOLOGIC PROFILE

General Use:

Treatment of hypertension of many causes, most commonly essential hypertension. Parenteral products are used in the treatment of hypertensive emergencies. Oral treatment should be initiated as soon as possible and individualized to ensure compliance for long-term therapy. Therapy is initiated with agents having minimal side effects. When such therapy fails, more potent drugs with different side effects are added in an effort to control blood pressure while causing minimal patient discomfort.

General Action and Information:

As a group, the antihypertensives are used to lower blood pressure to a normal level (<90 mm Hg diastolic) or to the lowest level tolerated. The goal of antihypertensive therapy is prevention of end-organ damage. Antihypertensives are classified into groups according to their site of

---

*Because of space limitations, additional classes or drugs not represented in *Davis's Drug Guide for Nurses*, 7th edition, are provided in this *Pocket Companion*.

action. These include peripherally acting antiadrenergics; centrally acting alpha adrenergics; beta-adrenergic blockers; vasodilators; ACE inhibitors; angiotensin II antagonists; calcium channel blockers; diuretics; and indapamide, a diuretic with vasodilatory properties. Hypertensive emergencies may be managed with parenteral vasodilators such as nitroprusside or enalaprilat.

Contraindications:

Hypersensitivity to individual agents.

Precautions:

Choose agents carefully in pregnancy, during lactation, or in patients receiving cardiac glycosides. ACE inhibitors and angiotensin II antagonists should be avoided during pregnancy. Alpha-adrenergic agonists and beta-adrenergic blockers should be used only in patients who will comply, because abrupt discontinuation of these agents may result in rapid and excessive rise in blood pressure (rebound phenomenon). Thiazide diuretics may increase the requirement for insulin, diet therapy, or oral hypoglycemic agents in diabetcs. Vasodilators may cause tachycardia if used alone and are commonly used in combination with beta-adrenergic blocking agents. Most antihypertensives (except for beta-adrenergic blockers, ACE inhibitors, angiotensin II receptor antagonists, and calcium channel blockers) cause sodium and water retention and are usually combined with a diuretic.

Interactions:

Many drugs can negate the therapeutic effectiveness of antihypertensives, including antihistamines, NSAIDs, sympathomimetic bronchodilators, decongestants, appetite suppressants, antidepressants, and MAO inhibitors. Hypokalemia from diuretics may increase the risk of cardiac glycoside toxicity. Potassium supplements and potassium-sparing diuretics may cause hyperkalemia when used with ACE inhibitors.

NURSING IMPLICATIONS

Assessment

- Monitor blood pressure and pulse frequently during dosage adjustment and periodically throughout therapy.
- Monitor intake and output ratios and daily weight.
- Monitor frequency of prescription refills to determine compliance.

Potential Nursing Diagnoses

- Tissue perfusion, altered (Indications).
- Knowledge deficit, related to medication regimen (Patient/Family Teaching).
- Noncompliance (Patient/Family Teaching).

Implementation

- Many antihypertensive agents are available as combination products to enhance compliance (see Appendix B).

Patient/Family Teaching

- Instruct patient to continue taking medication, even if feeling well. Abrupt withdrawal may cause rebound hypertension. Medication controls but does not cure hypertension.
- Encourage patient to comply with additional interventions for hypertension (weight reduction, low-sodium diet, regular exercise, discontinuation of smoking, moderation of alcohol consumption, and stress management).
- Instruct patient and family on proper technique for monitoring blood pressure. Advise them to check blood pressure weekly and report significant changes.
- Caution patient to make position changes slowly to minimize orthostatic hypotension. Advise patient that exercise or hot weather may enhance hypotensive effects.
- Advise patient to consult health care professional before taking any OTC medications, especially cold remedies.
- Advise patient to inform health care professional of medication regimen before treatment or surgery.
- Patients taking ACE inhibitors or angiotensin II antagonists should notify health care professional if pregnancy is planned or suspected.
- Emphasize the importance of follow-up exams to monitor progress.

Evaluation

Effectiveness of therapy can be demonstrated by: ■ Decrease in blood pressure.

Antihypertensive Agents Included in *Davis's Drug Guide for Nurses*

alpha-adreneric blocking agent
phenoxybenzamine 1179

angiotensin-converting enzyme (ACE) inhibitors
benazepril 63
captopril 63
enalapril, enalaprilat 63
fosinopril 64
lisinopril 64
moexipril 64
perindopril 64
quinapril 64
ramipril 64
trandolapril 64

angiotension II antagonists
candesartan 61
irbesartan 61
losartan 61
valsartan 61

beta-adrenergic blocking agents
acebutolol 1
atenolol 79
betaxolol 100
carteolol 160
carvedilol 162

labetalol 555
metoprolol 638
nadolol 678
penbutolol 758
pindolol 799
propranolol 849
timolol 996

calcium channel blockers
amlodipine 41
diltiazem 293
felodipine 384
isradipine 541
nicardipine 699
nifedipine 705
nisoldipine 711
verapamil 1037

centrally acting adrenergics
clonidine 212
guanabenz 455
guanfacine 459
methyldopa P-96

diuretics
chlorothiazide 315
chlorthalidone 315
furosemide 308

*Because of space limitations, additional classes or drugs not represented in *Davis's Drug Guide for Nurses*, 7th edition, are provided in this *Pocket Companion*.

hydrochlorthiazide 308
indapamide 512
metolazone 636
torsemide 308

peripherally acting antiadrenergics
doxazosin 328
guanadrel 457

prazosin 825
terazosin 960

vasodilators
hydralazine 481
minoxidil 652
nitroprusside 717

ANTI-INFECTIVE AGENTS

PHARMACOLOGIC PROFILE

General Use:

Treatment and prophylaxis of various bacterial infections. See specific drugs for spectrum and indications. Some infections may require additional surgical intervention and supportive therapy.

General Action and Information:

Kill (bactericidal) or inhibit the growth of (bacteriostatic) susceptible pathogenic bacteria. Not active against viruses or fungi. Anti-infective agents are subdivided into categories depending on chemical similarities and antimicrobial spectrum.

Contraindications:

Known hypersensitivity to individual agents. Cross-sensitivity among related agents may occur.

Precautions:

Culture and susceptibility testing are desirable to optimize therapy. Dosage modification may be required in patients with hepatic or renal insufficiency. Use cautiously in pregnant and lactating women. Prolonged inappropriate use of broad spectrum anti-infective agents may lead to superinfection with fungi or resistant bacteria.

Interactions:

Penicillins and aminoglycosides chemically inactivate each other and should not be physically admixed. Erythromycins may decrease hepatic metabolism of other drugs. Probenecid increases serum levels of penicillins and related compounds. Highly protein-bound anti-infectives such as sulfonamides may displace or be displaced by other highly bound drugs. See individual drugs. Extended-spectrum penicillins (ticarcillin, piperacillin) and some cephalosporins (cefamandole, cefoperazone, cefotetan) may increase the risk of bleeding with anticoagulants, antiplatelet agents, or NSAIDs. Fluoroquinolone absorption is decreased by antacids, bismuth subsalicylate, iron salts, sucralfate, and zinc salts.

NURSING IMPLICATIONS

Assessment

- Assess patient for signs and symptoms of infection prior to and throughout therapy.
- Determine previous hypersensitivities in patients receiving penicillins or cephalosporins.
- Obtain specimens for culture and sensitivity prior to initiating therapy. First dose may be given before receiving results.

Potential Nursing Diagnoses

- Infection, risk for (Indications).
- Knowledge deficit, related to medication regimen (Patient/Family Teaching).
- Noncompliance (Patient/Family Teaching).

Implementation

- Most anti-infectives should be administered around the clock to maintain therapeutic serum drug levels.

Patient/Family Teaching

- Instruct patient to continue taking medication around the clock until finished completely, even if feeling better.
- Advise patient to report the signs of superinfection (black, furry overgrowth on the tongue; vaginal itching or discharge; loose or foul-smelling stools) and allergy to health care professional.
- Instruct patient to notify health care professional if fever and diarrhea develop, especially if stool contains pus, blood, or mucus. Advise patient not to treat diarrhea without consulting health care professional.
- Instruct patient to notify health care professional if symptoms do not improve.

Evaluation

Effectiveness of therapy can be demonstrated by: ■ Resolution of the signs and symptoms of infection. Length of time for complete resolution depends on organism and site of infection.

Anti-infective Agents Included in *Davis's Drug Guide for Nurses*

aminoglycosides
amikacin 30
gentamicin 30
kanamycin 30
neomycin 30
netilmicin 30
streptomycin 30
tobramycin 30

antimalarial
quinine P–103

antiprotozoal
pentamide 771

carbapenem
imipenem/cilastatin 507

cephalosporins—first generation
cefadroxil 167
cefazolin 167
cephalexin 167
cephapirin 167

cephradine 167

cephalosporins—second generation
cefaclor 171
cefamandole 171
cefmetazole 171
cefonicid 171
cefotetan 171
cefoxitin 171
cefprozil 171
cefuroxime 171
loracarbef 171

cephalosporins—third generation
cefdinir 176
cefepime 176
cefixime 176
cefoperazone 176
cefotaxime 177
cefpodixime 177
ceftazidime 177
ceftibuten 177

---

*Because of space limitations, additional classes or drugs not represented in *Davis's Drug Guide for Nurses*, 7th edition, are provided in this *Pocket Companion*.

ceftizoxime 177
ceftriaxone 177

extended-spectrum penicillins
piperacillin 802
piperacillin/tazobactam 802
ticarcillin 990
ticarcillin/clavulanate 990

fluoroquinolones
alatrovafloxacin 408
ciprofloxacin 408
enoxacin 408
gatifloxacin 408
levofloxacin 408
lomefloxacin 408
moxifloxacin 408
norfloxacin 408
ofloxacin 408
sparfloxacin 408
trovafloxacin 408

macrolides
azithromycin 87
clarithromycin 204
erythromycin 360

penicillins
amoxicillin 43
amoxicillin/clavulanate 45
ampicillin 51
ampicillin/sulbactam 54
benzathine penicillin G 764
penicillin G potassium 764

procaine penicillin G 764
penicillin G sodium 764
penicillin V 764

penicillinase-resistant penicillins
cloxacillin 767
dicloxacillin 767
methicillin 767
nafcillin 767
oxacillin 767

sulfonamides
sulfacetamide 1158
sulfamethoxazole 942
trimethoprim/sulfamethoxazole 1025

tetracyclines
demeclocyline 1173
doxycycline 969
minocycline 969
tetracycline 969

miscellaneous
bacitracin 1171
chloramphenicol 1157
clindamycin 206
dapsone 1173
immune globulin 879
metronidazole 641
nitrofurantoin 712
silver sulfadiazine 1181
trimethoprim 1024
vancomycin 1033

ANTINEOPLASTIC AGENTS

PHARMACOLOGIC AGENTS

General Use:

Used in the treatment of various solid tumors, lymphomas, and leukemias. Also used in some autoimmune disorders such as rheumatoid arthritis (cyclophosphamide, methotrexate). Often used in combinations to minimize individual toxicities and increase response. Chemotherapy may be combined with other treatment modalities such as surgery and radiation therapy. Dosages vary greatly, depending on extent of disease, other agents used, and patient's condition. Some new formulations (daunorubicin, doxorubicin) encapsulated in a lipid membrane have less toxicity with greater efficacy.

General Action and Information:

Act by many different mechanisms (see the following table). Most commonly affect DNA synthesis or function. Action may not be limited to neoplastic cells.

MECHANISM OF ACTION OF VARIOUS ANTINEOPLASTIC AGENTS

MECHANISM OF ACTION	AGENT	EFFECTS ON CELL CYCLE
ALKYLATING AGENTS Cause cross-linking of DNA	busulfan carboplatin chlorambucil cisplatin cyclophosphamide dacarbazine ifosfamide mechlorethamine melphalan procarbazine temozolamide thiotepa	Cell cycle–nonspecific
ANTHRACYCLINES Interfere with DNA and RNA synthesis	daunorubicin doxorubicin idarubicin	Cell cycle–nonspecific
ANTIMETABOLITES Take the place of normal proteins	capecitabine cytarabine fluorouracil fludarabine hydroxyurea mercaptopurine methotrexate	Cell cycle–specific, work mostly in S phase (DNA synthesis)
ANTITUMOR ANTIBIOTICS Interfere with DNA and RNA synthesis	bleomycin dactinomycin mitomycin mitoxantrone plicamycin streptozocin	Cell cycle–nonspecific (except bleomycin)
ENZYMES Depletes asparagine	asparaginase pegaspargase	Cell-cycle phase–specific
ENZYME INHIBITORS Inhibit topoisomerase	irinotecan topotecan	Cell-cycle phase–specific
HORMONAL AGENTS Alter hormonal status in tumors that are sensitive	bicalutamide estramustine flutamide leuprolide megestrol nilutamide tamoxifen testosterone (androgens)	Unknown
HORMONAL AGENTS–AROMATASE INHIBITORS Inhibit enzyme responsible for activating estrogen	anastrazole letrozole	Unknown
IMMUNE MODULATORS	aldesleukin BCG trastuzumab	Unknown
PODOPHYLLOTOXIN DERIVATIVES Damages DNA before mitosis	etoposide tenoposide	Cell-cycle phase–specific
TAXOIDS Interupt interphase and mitosis	docetaxel paclitaxel	Cell-cycle phase–specific
VINCA ALKALOIDS Interfere with mitosis	vinblastine vincristine vinorelbine	Cell cycle–specific, work during M phase (mitosis)
MISCELLANEOUS	aldesleukin altretamine	Unknown Unknown

Contraindications:

Previous bone marrow depression or hypersensitivity. Contraindicated in pregnancy and lactation.

---

*Because of space limitations, additional classes or drugs not represented in *Davis's Drug Guide for Nurses*, 7th edition, are provided in this *Pocket Companion*.

Precautions:

Use cautiously in patients with active infections, decreased bone marrow reserve, radiation therapy, or other debilitating illnesses. Use cautiously in patients with childbearing potential.

Interactions:

Allopurinol decreases metabolism of mercaptopurine. Toxicity from methotrexate may be increased by other nephrotoxic drugs or larger doses of aspirin or NSAIDs. Bone marrow depression is additive. See individual drugs.

NURSING IMPLICATIONS

Assessment

- Monitor for bone marrow depression. Assess for bleeding (bleeding gums, bruising, petechiae, guaiac stools, urine, and emesis) and avoid IM injections and rectal temperatures if platelet count is low. Apply pressure to venipuncture sites for 10 min. Assess for signs of infection during neutropenia. Anemia may occur. Monitor for increased fatigue, dyspnea, and orthostatic hypotension.
- Monitor intake and output ratios, appetite, and nutritional intake. Prophylactic antiemetics may be used. Adjusting diet as tolerated may help maintain fluid and electrolyte balance and nutritional status.
- Monitor IV site carefully and ensure patency. Discontinue infusion immediately if discomfort, erythema along vein, or infiltration occurs. Tissue ulceration and necrosis may result from infiltration.
- Monitor for symptoms of gout (increased uric acid, joint pain, and edema). Encourage patient to drink at least 2 liters of fluid each day. Allopurinol may be given to decrease uric acid levels. Alkalinization of urine may be ordered to increase excretion of uric acid.

Potential Nursing Diagnoses

- Infection, risk for (Side Effects).
- Nutrition, altered: less than body requirements (Adverse Reactions).
- Knowledge deficit, related to medication regimen (Patient/Family Teaching).

Implementation

- Solutions for injection should be prepared in a biologic cabinet. Wear gloves, gown, and mask while handling medication. Discard equipment in designated containers (see Appendix J for guidelines for safe handling).
- Check dose carefully. Fatalities have resulted from dosing errors.

Patient/Family Teaching

- Caution patient to avoid crowds and persons with known infections. Health care professional should be informed immediately if symptoms of infection occur.
- Instruct patient to report unusual bleeding. Advise patient of thrombocytopenia precautions.
- These drugs may cause gonadal suppression; however, patient should still use birth control, as most antineoplastics are teratogenic. Advise patient to inform health care professional immediately if pregnancy is suspected.
- Discuss with patient the possibility of hair loss. Explore methods of coping.
- Instruct patient to inspect oral mucosa for erythema and ulceration. If ulceration occurs, advise patient to use sponge brush and to rinse mouth with water after eating and drinking.

Topical agents may be used if mouth pain interferes with eating. Stomatitis pain may require treatment with opioid analgesics.

- Instruct patient not to receive any vaccinations without advice of health care professional. Antineoplastics may decrease antibody response and increase risk of adverse reactions.
- Advise patient of need for medical follow-up and frequent lab tests.

Evaluation

Effectiveness of therapy can be demonstrated by: ■ Decrease in size and spread of tumor ■ Improvement in hematologic status in patients with leukemia.

Antineoplastic Agents Included in *Davis's Drug Guide for Nurses*

alkylating agents
busulfan 132
carboplatin 154
chlorambucil 186
cisplatin 199
cyclophosphamide 249
estramustine 1175
ifosfamide 505
mechlorethamine 602
melphalan 609
procarbazine 830
temozolamide 959
thiotepa 1182

anthracyclines
daunorubicin citrate liposome 265
daunorubicin hydrochloride 265
doxorubicin 332
doxorubicin hydrochloride liposome 333
idarubicin 502

antimetabolites
cytarabine 256
floxuridine 1176
fludarabine 1176
fluorouracil 414
hydroxyurea 491
metacaptorpurine 1178
methotrexate 627
thioguanine 1182

antitumor antibiotics
bleomycin 114
mitomycin 656
mitoxantrone 659
plicamycin 809
streptozocin 1182

enzymes
asparaginase 77

pegaspargase 754

enzyme inhibitors
irinotecan 530
pentostatin 1179
topotecan 1008

estrogen blockers
tamoxifen 954
toremifene 1010

hormones
bicalutamide 103
estramustine 1175
flutamide 425
leuprolide 570
megestrol 608
nilutamide 708
tamoxifen 954

hormones–aromatase inhibitors
anastrazole 60
letrozole 566

immune modifiers
aldesleukin 15
BCG-Connaught Strain 1171
BCG-Tice Strain 1171
trastuzumab 1013

podophyllotoxin derivatives
etoposide 380
teniposide 1152

taxoids
docetaxel 319
paclitaxel 743

vinca alkaloids
vinblastine 1040
vincristine 1042
vinorelbine 1045

---

*Because of space limitations, additional classes or drugs not represented in *Davis's Drug Guide for Nurses*, 7th edition, are provided in this *Pocket Companion*.

miscellaneous
aldesleukin 15
altretamine 24
masoprocol 1177

mitotane 1178
porfimer 1180
tretinion (oral) 1183

ANTIPARKINSON AGENTS

PHARMACOLOGIC PROFILE

General Use:

Used in the treatment of parkinsonism of various causes: degenerative, toxic, infective, neoplastic, or drug-induced.

General Action and Information:

Drugs used in the treatment of the parkinsonian syndrome and other dyskinesias are aimed at restoring the natural balance of two major neurotransmitters in the CNS: acetylcholine and dopamine. The imbalance is a deficiency in dopamine that results in excessive cholinergic activity. Drugs used are either anticholinergics (benztropine, biperiden, and trihexyphenidyl) or dopaminergic agonists (bromocriptine, levodopa, and pergolide). Pramipexole and ropinerole are two new nonergot dopamine agonists. Entacapone inhibits the enzyme that breaks down levodopa, thereby enhancing its effects.

Contraindications:

Anticholinergics should be avoided in patients with narrow-angle glaucoma.

Precautions:

Use cautiously in patients with severe cardiac disease, pyloric obstruction, or prostatic enlargement.

Interactions:

Pyridoxine, MAO inhibitors, benzodiazepines, phenytoin, phenothiazines, and haloperidol may antagonize the effects of levodopa. Agents that antagonize dopamine (phenothiazines, metoclopramide) may decrease effectiveness of dopamine agonists.

NURSING IMPLICATIONS

Assessment

- Assess parkinsonian and extrapyramidal symptoms (akinesia, rigidity, tremors, pill rolling, mask facies, shuffling gait, muscle spasms, twisting motions, and drooling) before and throughout course of therapy. On-off phenomenon may cause symptoms to appear or improve suddenly.
- Monitor blood pressure frequently during therapy. Instruct patient to remain supine during and for several hours after 1st dose of bromocriptine, as severe hypotension may occur.

Potential Nursing Diagnoses

- Physical mobility, impaired (Indications).
- Injury, risk for (Indications).
- Knowledge deficit, related to medication regimen (Patient/Family Teaching).

Implementation

- In the carbidopa/levodopa combination, the number following the drug name represents the milligram of each drug.

Patient/Family Teaching

- May cause drowsiness or dizziness. Advise patient to avoid driving or other activities that require alertness until response to medication is known.
- Caution patient to make position changes slowly to minimize orthostatic hypotension.
- Instruct patient that frequent rinsing of mouth, good oral hygiene, and sugarless gum or candy may decrease dry mouth. Patient should notify health care professional if dryness persists (saliva substitutes may be used). Also notify the dentist if dryness interferes with use of dentures.
- Advise patient to confer with health care professional before taking OTC medications, especially cold remedies, or drinking alcoholic beverages. Patients receiving levodopa should avoid multivitamins. Vitamin B_6 (pyridoxine) may interfere with levodopa's action.
- Caution patient that decreased perspiration may occur. Overheating may occur during hot weather. Patients should remain indoors in an air-conditioned environment during hot weather.
- Advise patient to increase activity, bulk, and fluid in diet to minimize constipating effects of medication.
- Advise patient to notify health care professional if confusion, rash, urinary retention, severe constipation, visual changes, or worsening of parkinsonian symptoms occur.

Evaluation

Effectiveness of therapy can be demonstrated by: ■ Resolution of parkinsonian signs and symptoms ■ Resolution of drug-induced extrapyramidal symptoms.

Antiparkinson Agents Included in *Davis's Drug Guide for Nurses*

anticholinergics
benztropine 96
biperiden 107
trihexyphenidyl 1021

catechol-O-methyltransferase inhibitor
entacapone 341

dopamine agonists
amantadine 1169
bromocriptine 116
carbidopa/levodopa 574
levodopa 574
pergolide 780
pramipexole 823
ropinirole 899

ANTIPLATELET AGENTS

PHARMACOLOGIC PROFILE

General Use:

Antiplatelet agents are used to treat and prevent thromboembolic events such as stroke and myocardial infarction. Dipyridamole is commonly used after cardiac surgery.

*Because of space limitations, additional classes or drugs not represented in *Davis's Drug Guide for Nurses*, 7th edition, are provided in this *Pocket Companion*.

General Action and Information:

Inhibit platelet aggregation, prolongs bleeding time, and are used to prevent myocardial infarction or stroke (aspirin, clopidogrel, dipyridamole, ticlopidine). Abciximab, eptifibatide, and tirofiban are used in the management of various acute coronary syndromes. These agents have been used concurrently/sequentially with anticoagulants and thrombolytic agents.

Contraindications:

Hypersensitivity, ulcer disease, active bleeding, and recent surgery.

Precautions:

Use cautiously in patients at risk for bleeding (trauma, surgery). History of GI bleeding or ulcer disease. Safety not established in pregnancy, lactation, or children.

Interactions:

Concurrent use with NSAIDs, heparin, thrombolytic agents, or warfarin may increase the risk of bleeding.

NURSING IMPLICATIONS

Assessment

- Assess patient taking anticoagulants for signs of bleeding and hemorrhage (bleeding gums; nosebleed; unusual bruising; tarry, black stools; hematuria; fall in hematocrit or blood pressure; guaiac-positive stools; urine; or nasogastric aspirate).
- Assess patient for evidence of additional or increased thrombosis. Symptoms will depend on area of involvement.
- Assess patient taking antiplatelet agents for symptoms of stroke, peripheral vascular disease, or myocardial infarction periodically throughout therapy.
- **Lab Test Considerations:** Monitor activated partial thromboplastin time (aPTT) or international normalized ratio (INR) with full-dose heparin therapy, prothrombin time (PT) with warfarin therapy, and hematocrit and other clotting factors frequently during therapy.
- Monitor bleeding time throughout antiplatelet therapy. Prolonged bleeding time, which is time- and dose-dependent, is expected.
- **Toxicity and Overdose:** If overdose occurs or anticoagulation needs to be immediately reversed, the antidote for heparins is protamine sulfate; for warfarin, the antidote is vitamin K (phytonadione [AquaMEPHYTON]). Administration of whole blood or plasma may also be required in severe bleeding due to warfarin because of the delayed onset of vitamin K.

Potential Nursing Diagnoses

- Tissue perfusion, altered (Indications).
- Injury, risk for (Side Effects).
- Knowledge deficit, related to medication regimen (Patient/Family Teaching).

Implementation

- Inform all personnel caring for patient of anticoagulant therapy. Venipunctures and injection sites require application of pressure to prevent bleeding or hematoma formation.
- Use an infusion pump with continuous infusions to ensure accurate dosage.

Patient/Family Teaching

- Caution patient to avoid activities leading to injury, to use a soft toothbrush and electric razor, and to report any symptoms of unusual bleeding or bruising to health care professional immediately.
- Instruct patient not to take OTC medications, especially those containing aspirin, NSAIDs, or alcohol, without advice of health care professional.
- Review foods high in vitamin K (see Appendix L) with patients on warfarin. Patient should have consistent limited intake of these foods, as vitamin K is the antidote for warfarin and greatly alternating intake of these foods will cause PT levels to fluctuate.
- Emphasize the importance of frequent lab tests to monitor coagulation factors.
- Instruct patient to carry identification describing medication regimen at all times and to inform all health care personnel caring for patient of anticoagulant therapy before laboratory tests, treatment, or surgery.

Evaluation

Effectiveness of therapy can be demonstrated by: ■ Prevention of undesired clotting and its sequelae without signs of hemorrhage ■ Prevention of stroke, myocardial infarction, and vascular death in patients at risk.

Antiplatelet Agents Included in *Davis's Drug Guide for Nurses*

abciximab 1168	eptifibatide 354
aspirin 903	ticlopidine 993
clopidogrel 215	tirofiban 998
dipyridamole 304	

ANTIPSYCHOTIC AGENTS

PHARMACOLOGIC PROFILE

General Use:

Treatment of acute and chronic psychoses, particularly when accompanied by increased psychomotor activity. Use of clozapine is limited to schizophrenia unresponsive to conventional therapy. Selected agents are also used as antihistamines or antiemetics. Chlorpromazine is also used in the treatment of intractable hiccups.

General Action and Information:

Block dopamine receptors in the brain; also alter dopamine release and turnover. Peripheral effects include anticholinergic properties and alpha-adrenergic blockade. Most antipsychotics are phenothiazines except for haloperidol, which is a butyrophenone, and clozapine, which is a miscellaneous compound. Newer agents such as olanzapine, quetiapine, and risperidone may have fewer adverse reactions. Phenothiazines differ in their ability to produce sedation (greatest with chlorpromazine and thioridazine), extrapyramidal reactions (greatest with prochlorperazine and trifluoperazine), and anticholinergic effects (greatest with chlorpromazine).

---

*Because of space limitations, additional classes or drugs not represented in *Davis's Drug Guide for Nurses*, 7th edition, are provided in this *Pocket Companion*.

Contraindications:

Hypersensitivity. Cross-sensitivity may exist among phenothiazines. Should not be used in narrow-angle glaucoma. Should not be used in patients who have CNS depression.

Precautions:

Safety in pregnancy and lactation not established. Use cautiously in patients with symptomatic cardiac disease. Avoid exposure to extremes in temperature. Use cautiously in severely ill or debilitated patients, diabetics, and patients with respiratory insufficiency, prostatic hypertrophy, or intestinal obstruction. May lower seizure threshold. Clozapine may cause agranulocytosis. Most agents are capable of causing neuroleptic malignant syndrome.

Interactions:

Additive hypotension with acute ingestion of alcohol, antihypertensives, or nitrates. Antacids may decrease absorption. Phenobarbital may increase metabolism and decrease effectiveness. Additive CNS depression with other CNS depressants, including alcohol, antihistamines, antidepressants, opioid analgesics, or sedative/hypnotics. Lithium may decrease blood levels and effectiveness of phenothiazines. May decrease the therapeutic response to levodopa. May increase the risk of agranulocytosis with antithyroid agents.

NURSING IMPLICATIONS

Assessment

- Assess patient's mental status (orientation, mood, behavior) before and periodically throughout therapy.
- Monitor blood pressure (sitting, standing, lying), pulse, and respiratory rate before and frequently during the period of dosage adjustment.
- Observe patient carefully when administering medication to ensure medication is actually taken and not hoarded.
- Monitor patient for onset of *akathisia* (restlessness or desire to keep moving) and extrapyramidal side effects (*parkinsonian*—difficulty speaking or swallowing, loss of balance control, pill rolling, mask-like face, shuffling gait, rigidity, tremors; and *dystonia*—muscle spasms, twisting motions, twitching, inability to move eyes, weakness of arms or legs) every 2 mo during therapy and 8–12 wk after therapy has been discontinued. Parkinsonian effects are more common in geriatric patients and dystonias are more common in younger patients. Notify health care professional if these symptoms occur, as reduction in dosage or discontinuation of medication may be necessary. Trihexyphenidyl or diphenhydramine may be used to control these symptoms.
- Monitor for *tardive dyskinesia* (uncontrolled rhythmic movement of mouth, face, and extremities; lip smacking or puckering; puffing of cheeks; uncontrolled chewing; rapid or worm-like movements of tongue). Notify health care professional immediately if these symptoms occur; these side effects may be irreversible.
- Monitor for development of *neuroleptic malignant syndrome* (fever, respiratory distress, tachycardia, convulsions, diaphoresis, hypertension or hypotension, pallor, tiredness, severe muscle stiffness, loss of bladder control.) Notify health care professional immediately if these symptoms occur.

Potential Nursing Diagnoses

- Thought processes, altered (Indications).
- Knowledge deficit, related to medication regimen (Patient/Family Teaching).

■ Noncompliance (Patient/Family Teaching).

Implementation

■ **General Info:** Keep patient recumbent for at least 30 min following parenteral administration to minimize hypotensive effects.
■ To prevent contact dermatitis, avoid getting solution on hands.
■ Phenothiazines should be discontinued 48 hr before and not resumed for 24 hr following myelography, as they lower the seizure threshold.
■ **PO:** Administer with food, milk, or a full glass of water to minimize gastric irritation.
■ Dilute most concentrates in 120 ml of distilled or acidified tap water or fruit juice just before administration.

Patient/Family Teaching

■ Advise patient to take medication exactly as directed and not to skip doses or double up on missed doses. Abrupt withdrawal may lead to gastritis, nausea, vomiting, dizziness, headache, tachycardia, and insomnia.
■ Advise patient to make position changes slowly to minimize orthostatic hypotension.
■ Medication may cause drowsiness. Caution patient to avoid driving or other activities requiring alertness until response to the medication is known.
■ Caution patient to avoid taking alcohol or other CNS depressants concurrently with this medication.
■ Advise patient to use sunscreen and protective clothing when exposed to the sun to prevent photosensitivity reactions. Extremes of temperature should also be avoided, as these drugs impair body temperature regulation.
■ Advise patient that increasing activity, bulk, and fluids in the diet helps minimize the constipating effects of this medication.
■ Instruct patient to use frequent mouth rinses, good oral hygiene, and sugarless gum or candy to minimize dry mouth.
■ Advise patient to notify health care professional of medication regimen before treatment or surgery.
■ Emphasize the importance of routine follow-up exams and continued participation in psychotherapy as indicated.

Evaluation

Effectiveness of therapy can be demonstrated by: ■ Decrease in excitable, paranoic, or withdrawn behavior ■ Relief of nausea and vomiting ■ Relief of intractable hiccups.

Antipsychotic Agents Included in *Davis's Drug Guide for Nurses*

butyrophenone
haloperidol 463

phenothiazines
chlorpromazine 191
fluphenazine 419
prochlorperazine 833
thioridazine 978
trifluoperazine 1018

---

*Because of space limitations, additional classes or drugs not represented in *Davis's Drug Guide for Nurses*, 7th edition, are provided in this *Pocket Companion*.

miscellaneous

clozapine 218

olanzapine 725

quetiapine 867

risperidone 891

ANTIPYRETIC AGENTS

PHARMACOLOGIC PROFILE

General Use:

Used to lower fever of many causes (infection, inflammation, and neoplasms).

General Action and Information:

Antipyretics lower fever by affecting thermoregulation in the CNS and by inhibiting the action of prostaglandins peripherally. Aspirin has the most profound effect on platelet function as compared with other salicylates, ibuprofen, or ketoprofen.

Contraindications:

Avoid aspirin, ibuprofen, or ketoprofen in patients with bleeding disorders (risk of bleeding is less with other salicylates). Aspirin and other salicylates should be avoided in children and adolescents.

Precautions:

Use aspirin, ibuprofen, or ketoprofen cautiously in patients with ulcer disease. Avoid chronic use of large doses of acetaminophen.

Interactions:

Large doses of aspirin may displace other highly protein-bound drugs. Additive GI irritation with aspirin, ibuprofen, ketoprofen, and other NSAIDs or corticosteroids. Aspirin, ibuprofen, ketoprofen, or naproxen may increase the risk of bleeding with other agents affecting hemostasis (anticoagulants, thrombolytics, antineoplastics, and certain anti-infectives).

NURSING IMPLICATIONS

Assessment

■ Assess fever; note presence of associated symptoms (diaphoresis, tachycardia, and malaise).

Potential Nursing Diagnoses

■ Body temperature, altered, risk for (Indications).

■ Knowledge deficit, related to medication regimen (Patient/Family Teaching).

Implementation

■ Administration with food or antacids may minimize GI irritation (aspirin, ibuprofen, ketoprofen, naproxen).

■ Available in oral and rectal dosage forms and in combination with other drugs.

Patient/Family Teaching

- Advise patient to consult health care professional if fever is not relieved by routine doses or if greater than 39.5°C (103°F) or lasts longer than 3 days.
- Centers for Disease Control and Prevention warns against giving aspirin to children or adolescents with varicella (chickenpox) or influenza-like or viral illnesses because of a possible association with Reye's syndrome.

Evaluation

Effectiveness of therapy can be demonstrated by: ■ Reduction of fever.

Antipyretic Agents Included in *Davis's Drug Guide for Nurses*

acetaminophen 3

aspirin 903

choline and magnesium salicylates 903

choline salicylate 903

ibuprofen 499

ketoprofen 550

salsalate 903

ANTIRETROVIRAL AGENTS

PHARMACOLOGIC PROFILE

General Use:

The goal of antiretroviral therapy in the management of HIV infection is to improve CD4 cell counts and decrease viral load. If accomplished, this generally results in slowed progression of the disease, improved quality of life, and decreased opportunistic infections. Perinatal use of agents also prevents transmission of the virus to the fetus. Postexposure prophylaxis with antiretrovirals is also recommended.

General Action and Information:

Because of the rapid emergence of resistance and toxicities of individual agents, HIV infection is almost always managed by a combination of agents. Selections and doses are based on individual toxicities, underlying organ system disease, concurrent drug therapy, and severity of illness. Various combinations are used; up to four agents may be used simultaneously. More than 100 agents are currently being tested in addition to those already approved by the Food and Drug Administration (FDA).

Contraindications:

Hypersensitivity. Because of highly varying toxicities among agents, see individual monographs for more specific information.

Precautions

Many agents require modification for renal impairment. Protease inhibitors may cause hyperglycemia and should be used cautiously in patients with diabetes. Hemophiliacs may also be at risk of bleeding when taking protease inhibitors. See individual monographs for specific information.

---

*Because of space limitations, additional classes or drugs not represented in *Davis's Drug Guide for Nurses*, 7th edition, are provided in this *Pocket Companion*.

Interactions:

There are many signficant interactions among the antiretrovirals. They are affected by drugs that alter metabolism; some agents themselves affect metabolism. See individual agents.

NURSING IMPLICATIONS

Assessment

- Assess patient for change in severity of symptoms of HIV and for symptoms of opportunistic infections throughout therapy.
- **Lab Test Considerations:** Monitor viral load and CD4 counts prior to and periodically during therapy.

Potential Nursing Diagnoses

- Infection, risk for (Indications).
- Knowledge deficit, related to medication regimen (Patient/Family Teaching).
- Noncompliance (Patient/Family Teaching).

Implementation

- Administer doses around the clock.

Patient/Family Teaching

- Instruct patient to take medication exactly as directed, around the clock, even if sleep is interrupted. Emphasize the importance of complying with therapy, not taking more than prescribed amount, and not discontinuing without consulting health care professional. Missed doses should be taken as soon as remembered unless almost time for next dose; patient should not double doses. Inform patient that long-term effects are unknown at this time.
- Instruct patient that antiretrovirals should not be shared with others.
- Inform patient that antiretroviral therapy does not cure HIV and does not reduce the risk of transmission of HIV to others through sexual contact or blood contamination. Caution patient to use a condom during sexual contact and to avoid sharing needles or donating blood to prevent spreading the AIDS virus to others.
- Advise patient to avoid taking any Rx or OTC medications without consulting health care professional.
- Emphasize the importance of regular follow-up exams and blood counts to determine progress and monitor for side effects.

Evaluation

Effectiveness of therapy can be demonstrated by: ■ Decrease in viral load and increase in CD4 counts in patients with HIV.

Antiretroviral Agents Included in *Davis's Drug Guide for Nurses*

non-nucleoside reverse transcriptase inhibitors	*nucleoside reverse transcriptase inhibitors*
delavirdine 270	didanosine 284
efavirenz 339	lamivudine 559
nevirapine 695	stavudine 937
	zalcitabine 1062

zidovudine 1066

protease inhibitors
indinavir 514

nelfinavir 691
ritonavir 894
saquinavir 909

ANTITHYROID AGENTS

PHARMACOLOGIC PROFILE

General Use:

Used in the treatment of hyperthyroidism of various causes (Graves' disease, multinodular goiter, thyroiditis, and thyrotoxic crisis) in children, pregnant women, and other patients in whom hyperthyroidism is not expected to be permanent. These agents are also used to prepare patients for thyroidectomy or for patients in whom thyroidectomy is contraindicated. Beta-adrenergic blockers (propranolol) are sometimes used in conjunction with antithyroid agents to control symptoms (tachycardia and tremor) but have no effect on thyroid status. Iodine and iodides are also used as radiation protectants.

General Action and Information:

Inhibit thyroid hormone formation (iodine) or inhibit oxidation of iodine (methimazole and propylthiouracil).

Contraindications:

Hypersensitivity. Previous bone marrow depression.

Precautions:

Use methimazole cautiously in patients with decreased bone marrow reserve.

Interactions:

Lithium may cause thyroid abnormalities and interfere with the response to antithyroid therapy. Phenothiazines may increase the risk of agranulocytosis.

NURSING IMPLICATIONS

Assessment

- **General Info:** Monitor response of symptoms of hyperthyroidism or thyrotoxicosis (tachycardia, palpitations, nervousness, insomnia, fever, diaphoresis, heat intolerance, tremors, weight loss, diarrhea).
- Assess patient for development of hypothyroidism (intolerance to cold, constipation, dry skin, headache, listlessness, tiredness, or weakness). Dosage adjustment may be required.
- Assess patient for skin rash or swelling of cervical lymph nodes. Treatment may be discontinued if this occurs.
- Monitor thyroid function studies before and periodically throughout therapy.
- **Iodides:** Assess for signs and symptoms of iodism (metallic taste, stomatitis, skin lesions, cold symptoms, severe GI upset) or anaphylaxis. Report these symptoms promptly to physician or other health care provider.

---

*Because of space limitations, additional classes or drugs not represented in *Davis's Drug Guide for Nurses*, 7th edition, are provided in this *Pocket Companion*.

Potential Nursing Diagnoses

■ Knowledge deficit, related to medication regimen (Patient/Family Teaching).

Implementation

■ Mix iodide solutions in a full glass of fruit juice, water, or milk. Administer after meals to minimize GI irritation.

Patient/Family Teaching

■ Instruct patient to take medication exactly as directed. Missing doses may precipitate hyperthyroidism.
■ Advise patient to consult health care professional regarding dietary sources of iodine (iodized salt, shellfish, cabbage, kale, turnips).
■ Advise patient to carry identification describing medication regimen at all times and to notify health care professional of medical regimen before treatment or surgery.
■ Emphasize the importance of routine exams to monitor progress and check for side effects.

Evaluation

Effectiveness of therapy can be demonstrated by: ■ Decrease in severity of symptoms of hyperthyroidism ■ Decrease in vascularity and friability of the thyroid gland before preparation for surgery ■ Protection of the thyroid gland during radiation emergencies.

Antithyroid Agents Included in *Davis's Drug Guide for Nurses*

methimazole 624
potassium iodide, saturated solution 525

propylthiouracil 853
strong iodine solution 525

ANTITUBERCULAR AGENTS

PHARMACOLOGIC PROFILE

General Use:

Used in the treatment and prevention of tuberculosis and diseases caused by other mycobacteria, including *Mycobacterium avium* complex (MAC), seen mostly in HIV patients. Combinations are used in the treatment of active disease tuberculosis to rapidly decrease the infectious state and delay or prevent the emergence of resistant strains. In selected situations, intermittent (twice weekly) regimens may be employed. Streptomycin is also used as an antitubercular agent. The anti-infective agents, azithromycin and clarithromycin, are useful in the prevention and management of MAC disease. Rifampin is used in the prevention of meningococcal meningitis and *Haemophilus influenzae* type b disease.

General Action and Information:

Kill (tuberculocidal) or inhibit the growth of (tuberculostatic) mycobacteria responsible for causing tuberculosis. Combination therapy with two or more agents is required, unless used as prophylaxis (isoniazid alone).

Contraindications:

Hypersensitivity. Severe liver disease.

Precautions:

Use cautiously in patients with a history of liver disease or in elderly or debilitated patients. Ethambutol requires ophthalmologic follow-up. Safety in pregnancy and lactation not established, although selected agents have been used without adverse effects on the fetus. Compliance is required for optimal response.

Interactions:

Isoniazid inhibits the metabolism of phenytoin. Rifampin significantly decreases saquinavir levels (combination should be avoided).

NURSING IMPLICATIONS

Assessment

- Mycobacterial studies and susceptibility tests should be performed prior to and periodically throughout therapy to detect possible resistance.
- Assess lung sounds and character and amount of sputum periodically throughout therapy.

Potential Nursing Diagnoses

- Infection, risk for (Indications).
- Knowledge deficit, related to medication regimen (Patient/Family Teaching).
- Noncompliance (Patient/Family Teaching).

Implementation

- Most medications can be administered with food or antacids if GI irritation occurs.

Patient/Family Teaching

- Advise patient of the importance of continuing therapy even after symptoms have subsided.
- Emphasize the importance of regular follow-up examinations to monitor progress and check for side effects.
- Inform patients taking *rifampin* that saliva, sputum, sweat, tears, urine, and feces may become red-orange to red-brown and that soft contact lenses may become permanently discolored.

Evaluation

Effectiveness of therapy can be demonstrated by: ■ Resolution of the signs and symptoms of tuberculosis ■ Negative sputum cultures.

Antitubercular Agents Included in *Davis's Drug Guide for Nurses*

ethambutol 374
isoniazid 537
pyrazinamide 859

rifampin 886
rifapentine 888

---

*Because of space limitations, additional classes or drugs not represented in *Davis's Drug Guide for Nurses*, 7th edition, are provided in this *Pocket Companion*.

ANTITUSSIVE AGENTS

PHARMACOLOGIC PROFILE

General Use:

Used for the symptomatic relief of cough due to various causes, including viral upper respiratory infections. Not intended for chronic use.

General Action and Information:

Antitussives (codeine, dextromethorphan, diphenhydramine, hydrocodone, and hydromorphone) suppress cough by central mechanisms. Benzonatate decreases cough by a local anesthetic action. Productive cough should not be suppressed unless it interferes with sleeping or other activities of daily living. Increasing fluid intake probably serves as the best expectorant, decreasing the viscosity of secretions so that they may be more easily mobilized.

Contraindications:

Hypersensitivity.

Precautions:

Use cautiously in children. Should not be used for prolonged periods unless under the advice of a physician or other health care professional.

Interactions:

Centrally acting antitussives may have additive CNS depression with other CNS depressants.

NURSING IMPLICATIONS

Assessment

- Assess frequency and nature of cough, lung sounds, and amount and type of sputum produced.

Potential Nursing Diagnoses

- Airway clearance, ineffective (Indications).
- Knowledge deficit, related to medication regimen (Patient/Family Teaching).

Implementation

- Unless contraindicated, maintain fluid intake of 1500–2000 ml to decrease viscosity of bronchial secretions.

Patient/Family Teaching

- Instruct patient to cough effectively, sit upright, and take several deep breaths before attempting to cough.
- Advise patient to minimize cough by avoiding irritants (cigarette smoke, fumes, dust). Humidification of environmental air, frequent sips of water, and sugarless hard candy may also decrease the frequency of dry, irritating cough.

- Caution patient to avoid taking concurrent alcohol or CNS depressants.
- May cause dizziness or drowsiness. Caution patient to avoid driving or other activities requiring alertness until response to medication is known.
- Advise patient that any cough lasting over 1 wk or accompanied by fever, chest pain, persistent headache, or skin rash warrants medical attention.

Evaluation

Effectiveness of therapy can be demonstrated by: ■ Decrease in frequency and intensity of cough without eliminating patient's cough reflex.

Antitussive Agents Included in *Davis's Drug Guide for Nurses*

benzonatate 95
codeine 221
dextromethorphan 277

diphenhydramine 300
hydrocodone 483
hydromorphone 486

ANTI-ULCER AGENTS

PHARMACOLOGIC PROFILE

General Use:

Treatment and prophylaxis of peptic ulcer and gastric hypersecretory conditions such as Zollinger-Ellison syndrome. Histamine H_2-receptor antagonists and gastric and pump inhibitors are also used in the management of GERD.

General Action and Information:

Because a great majority of peptic ulcer disease may be traced to GI infection with the organism *Helicobacter pylori*, eradication of the organism decreases symptomatology and recurrence. Anti-infectives with significant activity against the organism include amoxicillin, clarithromycin, metronidazole, and tetracycline. Bismuth also has anti-infective activity against *H. pylori*. Regimens may include 2 anti-infectives plus a gastric acid–pump inhibitor (lansoprazole, omeprazole) or 3 anti-infectives or 3 anti-infectives plus a gastric acid–pump inhibitor.

---

*Because of space limitations, additional classes or drugs not represented in *Davis's Drug Guide for Nurses*, 7th edition, are provided in this *Pocket Companion*.

REGIMENS FOR ERADICATING *H. PYLORI*

REGIMEN	DOSING
omeprazole	40 mg once daily on 1st day, then 20 mg once daily for 2 wk
clarithomycine	500 mg 3 times daily for 2 wk
ranitidine bismuth citrate	400 mg twice daily for 4 wk
clarithromycin	500 mg 3 times daily for 2 wk
metronidazole	250 mg 4 times daily (at meals and bedtime) for 2 wk
tetracycline	500 mg 4 times daily (at meals and bedtime) for 2 wk
bismuth subsalicylate	525 mg 4 times daily (at meals and bedtime) for 2 wk
lansoprazole	30 mg daily for 2 wk
clarithromycin	500 mg twice daily for 2 wk
amoxicillin	1 g twice daily for for 2 wk
lansoprazole	30 mg daily for 2 wk
amoxicillin	1 g 3 times daily for for 2 wk

Other medications used in the management of gastric/duodenal ulcer disease are aimed at neutralizing gastric acid (antacids), decreasing acid secretion (histamine H_2 antagonists, lansoprazole, misoprostol, omeprazole), or protecting the ulcer surface from further damage (misoprostol, sucralfate). Histamine H_2-receptor antagonists (blockers) competitively inhibit the action of histamine at the H_2 receptor, located primarily in gastric parietal cells, resulting in inhibition of gastric acid secretion. Misoprostol decreases gastric acid secretion and increases production of protective mucus. Omeprazole and lansoprazole prevent the transport of hydrogen ions into the gastric lumen.

Contraindications:

Hypersensitivity.

Precautions:

Most histamine H_2 antagonists require dosage reduction in renal impairment and in elderly patients. Magnesium-containing antacids should be used cautiously in patients with renal impairment. Misoprostol should be used cautiously in women with childbearing potential.

Interactions:

Calcium and magnesium-containing antacids decrease the absorption of tetracycline and fluoroquinolones. Cimetidine inhibits the ability of the liver to metabolize several drugs, increasing the risk of toxicity from warfarin, tricyclic antidepressants, theophylline, metoprolol, phenytoin, propranolol, and lidocaine. Omeprazole decreases metabolism of phenytoin, diazepam, and warfarin. All agents that increase gastric pH will decrease the absorption of ketoconazole.

NURSING IMPLICATIONS

Assessment

- **General Info:** Assess patient routinely for epigastric or abdominal pain and frank or occult blood in the stool, emesis, or gastric aspirate.

- **Antacids:** Assess for heartburn and indigestion as well as the location, duration, character, and precipitating factors of gastric pain.
- **Histamine H₂ Antagonists:** Assess elderly and severely ill patients for confusion routinely. Notify physician or other health care professional promptly should this occur.
- **Misoprostol:** Assess women of childbearing age for pregnancy. Medication is usually begun on 2nd or 3rd day of menstrual period following a negative serum pregnancy test within 2 wk of beginning therapy.
- **Lab Test Considerations:** *Histamine H₂ antagonists* antagonize the effects of pentagastrin and histamine during gastric acid secretion test. Avoid administration during the 24 hr preceding the test.
- May cause false-negative results in skin tests using allergen extracts. These drugs should be discontinued 24 hr prior to the test.

Potential Nursing Diagnoses

- Pain (Indications).
- Knowledge deficit, related to medication regimen (Patient/Family Teaching).

Implementation

- **Antacids:** Antacids cause premature dissolution and absorption of enteric-coated tablets and may interfere with absorption of other oral medications. Separate administration of antacids and other oral medications by at least 1 hr.
- Shake liquid preparations well before pouring. Follow administration with water to ensure passage to stomach. Liquid and powder dosage forms are considered to be more effective than chewable tablets.
- Chewable tablets must be chewed thoroughly before swallowing. Follow with half a glass of water.
- Administer 1 and 3 hr after meals and at bedtime for maximum antacid effect.
- **Misoprostol:** Administer with meals and at bedtime to reduce the severity of diarrhea.
- **Pantoprazole, Rabeprazole, Omeprazole, and Lansoprazole:** Administer before meals, preferably in the morning. Capsules should be swallowed whole; do not open, crush, or chew.
- May be administered concurrently with antacids.
- **Sucralfate:** Administer on an empty stomach 1 hr before meals and at bedtime. Do not crush or chew tablets. Shake suspension well prior to administration. If nasogastric administration is required, consult pharmacist, as protein-binding properties of sucralfate have resulted in formation of a bezoar when administered with enteral feedings and other medications.

Patient/Family Teaching

- **General Info:** Instruct patient to take medication as directed for the full course of therapy, even if feeling better. If a dose is missed, it should be taken as soon as remembered but not if almost time for next dose. Do not double doses.
- Advise patient to avoid alcohol, products containing aspirin, NSAIDs, and foods that may cause an increase in GI irritation.
- Advise patient to report onset of black, tarry stools to the physician or other health care professional promptly.
- Inform patient that cessation of smoking may help prevent the recurrence of duodenal ulcers.

---

*Because of space limitations, additional classes or drugs not represented in *Davis's Drug Guide for Nurses*, 7th edition, are provided in this *Pocket Companion*.

- **Antacids:** Caution patient to consult health care professional before taking antacids for more than 2 wk or if problem is recurring. Advise patient to consult health care professional if relief is not obtained or if symptoms of gastric bleeding (black, tarry stools; coffee-ground emesis) occur.
- **Misoprostol:** Emphasize that sharing of this medication may be dangerous.
- Inform patient that misoprostol may cause spontaneous abortion. Women of childbearing age must be informed of this effect through verbal and written information and must use contraception throughout therapy. If pregnancy is suspected, the woman should stop taking misoprostol and immediately notify her health care professional.
- **Sucralfate:** Advise patient to continue with course of therapy for 4–8 wk, even if feeling better, to ensure ulcer healing.
- Advise patient that an increase in fluid intake, dietary bulk, and exercise may prevent drug-induced constipation.

Evaluation

Effectiveness of therapy can be demonstrated by: ■ Decrease in GI pain and irritation ■ Prevention of gastric irritation and bleeding. Healing of duodenal ulcers can be seen by x-rays or endoscopy. Therapy with histamine H_2 antagonists is continued for at least 6 wk after initial episode ■ Decreased symptoms of GERD ■ Increase in the pH of gastric secretions (antacids) ■ Prevention of gastric ulcers in patients receiving chronic NSAID therapy (misoprostol only).

Anti-ulcer Agents Included in *Davis's Drug Guide for Nurses*

antacids
aluminum hydroxide 26
magaldrate 591
magnesium hydroxide/aluminun hydroxide 591
sodium bicarbonate 926

anti-infectives
amoxicillin 43
bismuth subsalicylate 110
clarithromycin 204
metronidazole 641
tetracycline 969

gastric acid–pump inhibitors
lansoprazole 563
omeprazole 727
pantoprazole 751
rabeprazole 875

histamine H_2-receptor antagonists
cimetidine 472
famotidine 472
nizatidine 472
ranitidine 472

miscellaneous
misoprostol 655
sucralfate 941

ANTIVIRAL AGENTS

PHARMACOLOGIC PROFILE

General Use:

Acyclovir, famciclovir, and valacylovir are used in the management of herpesvirus infections. Acyclovir also is used in the management of chickenpox. Zanamivir is ued primarily in the prevention of influenza A viral infections. Cidofovir, ganciclovir, and foscarnet are used in the treatment of cytomegalovirus (CMV) retinitis.

General Action and Information:

Most agents inhibit viral replication.

Contraindications:

Previous hypersensitivity.

Precautions:

All exept zanamivir require dosage adjustment in renal impairment. Acyclovir may cause renal impairment. Acyclovir may cause CNS toxicity. Foscarnet increases risk of seizures.

Interactions:

Acyclovir may have additive CNS and nephrotoxicity with drugs causing similar adverse reactions.

NURSING IMPLICATIONS

Assessment

- **General Info:** Assess patient for signs and symptoms of infection before and throughout therapy.
- **Ophth:** Assess eye lesions before and daily during therapy.
- **Topical:** Assess lesions before and daily during therapy.

Potential Nursing Diagnoses

- Infection, risk for (Indications).
- Skin integrity, impaired (Indications).
- Knowledge deficit, related to medication regimen (Patient/Family Teaching).

Implementation

- Most systemic antiviral agents should be administered around the clock to maintain therapeutic serum drug levels.

Patient/Family Teaching

- Instruct patient to continue taking medication around the clock for full course of therapy, even if feeling better.
- Advise patient that antivirals and antiretrovirals do not prevent transmission to others. Precautions should be taken to prevent spread of virus.
- Instruct patient in correct technique for topical or ophthalmic preparations.
- Instruct patient to notify health care professional if symptoms do not improve.

Evaluation

Effectiveness of therapy can be demonstrated by: ■ Prevention or resolution of the signs and symptoms of viral infection. Length of time for complete resolution depends on organism and site of infection.

---

*Because of space limitations, additional classes or drugs not represented in *Davis's Drug Guide for Nurses*, 7th edition, are provided in this *Pocket Companion*.

Antiviral Agents Included in *Davis's Drug Guide for Nurses*

acyclovir 8	ganciclovir 436
amantadine 1169	rimantadine 1181
cidofovir 196	trifuradine 1158
famciclovir 383	valacyclovir 1029
foscarnet 430	zanamivir 1065

BRONCHODILATORS

PHARMACOLOGIC PROFILE

General Use:

Used in the treatment of reversible airway obstruction due to asthma or COPD. Recently revised recommendations for management of asthma recommend that rapid-acting inhaled beta-ago-nist bronchodilators (not salmeterol) be reserved as acute relievers of bronchospasm; repeated or chronic use indicates the need for additional long-term contol agents including inhaled corticosteroids, mast cell stabilizers, and long-acting bronchodilators (oral theophyl-line or beta-agonists) and leukotriene modifiers (montelukast, zafirlukast). The place of the new agent zafirlukast has not yet been established.[†]

General Action and Information:

Beta-adrenergic agonists (albuterol, epinephrine, isoproterenol, metaproterenol, pirbuterol, and terbutaline) produce bronchodilation by stimulating the production of cyclic adenosine monophosphate (cAMP). Newer agents (albuterol, metaproterenol, pirbuterol, and terbuta-line) are relatively selective for pulmonary (beta$_2$) receptors, whereas older agents produce cardiac stimulation (beta$_2$-adrenergic effects) in addition to bronchodilation. Onset of action allows use in management of acute attacks except for salmeterol, which has delayed onset. Phosphodiesterase inhibitors (aminophylline, dyphylline, oxtriphylline, and theophylline) inhibit the breakdown of cAMP. Ipratropium is an anticholinergic compound that produces bronchodilation by blocking the action of acetylcholine in the respiratory tract. Montelukast and zafirlukast are leukotriene modifiers. Leukotrienes are components of slow-reacting sub-stance of anaphylaxis A (SRS-A), which may be a cause of bronchospasm.

Contraindications:

Hypersensitivity to agents, preservatives (bisulfites), or propellants used in their formulation. Avoid use in uncontrolled cardiac arrhythmias.

Precautions:

Use cautiously in patients with diabetes, cardiovascular disease, or hyperthyroidism.

Interactions:

Therapeutic effectiveness may be antagonized by concurrent use of beta-adrenergic blocking agents. Additive sympathomimetic effects with other adrenergic (sympathetic) drugs, including vasopressors and decongestants. Cardiovascular effects may be potentiated by antidepressants and MAO inhibitors.

[†]Highlights of the Expert Panel Report 2: Guidelines for the diagnosis and management of asthma. NIH Publication No. 97-4051A. May 1997.

NURSING IMPLICATIONS

Assessment

- Assess blood pressure, pulse, respiration, lung sounds, and character of secretions before and throughout therapy.
- Patients with a history of cardiovascular problems should be monitored for ECG changes and chest pain.

Potential Nursing Diagnoses

- Airway clearance, ineffective (Indications).
- Activity intolerance (Indications).
- Knowledge deficit, related to medication regimen (Patient/Family Teaching).

Implementation

- Administer around the clock to maintain therapeutic plasma levels.

Patient/Family Teaching

- Emphasize the importance of taking only the prescribed dose at the prescribed time intervals.
- Encourage the patient to drink adequate liquids (2000 ml/day minimum) to decrease the viscosity of the airway secretions.
- Advise patient to avoid OTC cough, cold, or breathing preparations without consulting health care professional and to minimize intake of xanthine-containing foods or beverages (colas, coffee, and chocolate), as these may increase side effects and cause arrhythmias.
- Caution patient to avoid smoking and other respiratory irritants.
- Instruct patient on proper use of metered-dose inhaler (see Appendix I).
- Advise patient to contact health care professional promptly if the usual dose of medication fails to produce the desired results, symptoms worsen after treatment, or toxic effects occur.
- Patients using other inhalation medications and bronchodilators should be advised to use bronchodilator first and allow 5 min to elapse before administering the other medication, unless otherwise directed by health care professional.

Evaluation

Effectiveness of therapy can be demonstrated by: ■ Decreased bronchospasm ■ Increased ease of breathing.

Bronchodilators Included in *Davis's Drug Guide for Nurses*

beta-adrenergic agonists
albuterol 13
epinephrine 345
isoproterenol 1177
metaproterenol 617
pirbuterol 805
salmeterol 907
terbutaline 964

leukotriene antagonists
montelukast 664
zafirlukast 1061

phosphodiesterase inhibitors (xanthines)
aminophylline 120
dyphylline 120
oxtriphylline 120
theophylline 120

---

*Because of space limitations, additional classes or drugs not represented in *Davis's Drug Guide for Nurses*, 7th edition, are provided in this *Pocket Companion*.

anticholinergic agent   ipratropium 528

CARDIOTONIC AND INOTROPIC AGENTS*

PHARMACOLOGIC PROFILE

General Use:

Management of congestive heart failure or cardiac decompensation unresponsive to conventional therapy with cardiac glycosides, diuretics, or vasodilators. Also used during cardiac surgery.

General Action and Information:

Increase cardiac output mainly by direct myocardial effects and some peripheral vascular effects. Myocardial contractility is increased by inhibiting cyclic adenosine monophosphate (cAMP) phosphodiesterase, which increases intracellular cAMP.

Contraindications:

Hypersensivity. Avoid use in patients with hypertrophic cardiomyopathy.

Precautions:

Safety in pregnancy, lactation, and children not established.

Interactions:

Amrinone may produce excessive hypotension when given with disopyramide. Agents that cause hypokalemia, hypomagnesemia, or hypercalcemia increase the risk of cardiac glycoside toxicity. Bradycardia from beta blockers may be additive with digitalis glycosides. Quinidine increases serum digoxin levels.

NURSING IMPLICATIONS

Assessment

- Monitor blood pressure, pulse, and respiration before and periodically throughout therapy.
- Monitor intake and output ratios and daily weights. Assess patient for signs and symptoms of congestive heart failure (peripheral edema, rales/crackles, dyspnea, weight gain, jugular vein distentions) thoughout therapy.
- Before administering intial loading dose, determine if patient has taken any cardiac glycoside preparations inthe preceding 2–3 wk.
- **Lab Test Considerations:** Serum electrolyte levels, especially potassium, magnesium, and calcium, and renal and hepatic function should be evaluated periodically during therapy.
- **Toxicity and Overdose:** Patients taking digitalis glycosides should have serum levels measured regularly.

Potential Nursing Diagnoses

- Cardiac output, decreased (Indications).
- Knowledge deficit, related to medication regimen (Patient/Family Teaching).

Implementation

- Hypokalemia should be corrected before administration of amrinone, milrinone, digoxin, or digitoxin.
- Hypovelemia should be corrected with volume expanders before administrations.

Patient/Family Teaching

- Advise patient to notify health care professional if symptoms are not relieved or worsen.
- Instruct patient to notify nurse immediately if pain or discomfort at the insertion site occurs during IV administration.

Evaluation

Effectiveness of therapy can be demonstrated by: ■ Increased cardiac output ■ Decrease in severity of congestive heart failure. ■ Increased urine output.

Cardiotonic and Inotropic Agents Included in *Davis's Drug Guide for Nurses*

amrinone 58	dopamine 326
digoxin 2287	milrinone 650
dobutamine 317	

CENTRAL NERVOUS SYSTEM STIMULANTS*

PHARMACOLOGIC PROFILE

General Use:

CNS stimulants are used as an adjunct in the treatment of ADHD and in the treatment of narcolepsy.

General Action and Information:

CNS stimulation results in increased attention span in ADHD, increased motor activity, mental alertness, and decreased fatigue in narcoleptic patients.

Contraindications:

Hypersensitivity. Pregnancy or lactation. Should not be used in patients with psychiatric illness or chemical dependence.

Precautions:

Use cautiously in patients with cardiovascular disease, hypertension, diabetes, and seizure disorders.

Interactions:

Additive sympathomimetic effects with other adrenergic agents. Use with MAO inhibitors results in hypertensive crisis.

---

*Because of space limitations, additional classes or drugs not represented in *Davis's Drug Guide for Nurses*, 7th edition, are provided in this *Pocket Companion*.

NURSING IMPLICATIONS

Assessment

- Monitor blood pressure, pulse, and respiration before and periodically throughout therapy.
- In treatment of ADHD, monitor weight biweekly and inform prescriber of significant loss. Monitor height periodically in children; report growth inhibition.
- In narcolepsy, observe and document frequency of narcoleptic episodes.
- Assess attention span, motor, or vocal tics; impulse control; and interactions with others for children with ADHD.
- May produce a false sense of euphoria and well-being. Monitor and provide rest periods.
- These agents have a high dependence abuse potential. Tolerance to medication occurs rapidly; do not increase dose.

Potential Nursing Diagnoses

- Thought processes, altered (Side Effects).
- Sleep pattern disturbance (Side Effects).
- Knowledge deficit, related to medication regimen (Patient/Family Teaching).

Implementation

- Therapy should use the lowest possible dose.
- Sustained-release capsules should be swallowed whole; do not break, crush, or chew.
- Chewable tablets should be chewed thoroughly before swallowing.
- **ADHD:** When symptoms are under control, dose reduction or interruption of therapy may be possible during the summer, or may be given on each of the 5 school days, with medication-free days on weekends and holidays.

Patient/Family Teaching

- Instruct patient to take medication at least 6 hr before bedtime to avoid sleep disturbances
- Inform patient that the side effect of dry mouth can be minimized with frequent mouth rinses with water or by chewing sugarless gum or candies.
- Advise patient to avoid caffeine.
- Medication may impair judgment, cause dizziness or blurred vision. Advise patient to use caution when driving or during other activities requiring mental alertness.
- Instruct patient to inform health care professional if nervousness, restlessness, insomnia, anorexia, or dry mouth becomes severe.
- Inform patient that periodic holiday from the drug may be ordered to assess progress and decrease dependence.
- Advise the patient to take weight measurements twice weekly and report weight loss to health care professional.
- In children receiving the medication for ADHD, inform school nurse of regimen.
- In patients taking pemoline, instruct about signs of hepatitis and to report promptly to the health care professional if they occur.

Evaluation

Effectiveness of therapy can be demonstrated by: ■ Calming effect with decreased hyperactivity and prolonged attention span in children with ADHD ■ Decrease in the frequency of narcolepsy symptoms.

Central Nervous System Stimulants Included in *Davis's Drug Guide for Nurses*

amphetamine 1170   pemoline 756
methylphenidate 632

CHOLINERGIC AGENTS

PHARMACOLOGIC PROFILE

General Use:

Used in the treatment of nonobstructive urinary retention (bethanechol) and in the diagnosis and treatment (neostigmine and pyridostigmine) of myasthenia gravis. Cholinesterase inhibitors may be used to reverse nondepolarizing neuromuscular blocking agents.

General Action and Information:

Cholinergic agents intensify and prolong the action of acetylcholine by either mimicking its effects at cholinergic receptor sites (bethanechol) or preventing the breakdown of acetylcholine by inhibiting cholinesterases (neostigmine). Effects include increased tone in GU and skeletal muscle, decreased intraocular pressure, increased secretions, and decreased bladder capacity.

Contraindications:

Hypersensitivity. Avoid use in patients with possible obstruction of the GI or GU tract.

Precautions:

Use with extreme caution in patients with a history of asthma, peptic ulcer disease, cardiovascular disease, epilepsy, or hyperthyroidism. Safety in pregnancy and lactation not established. Atropine should be available to treat excessive dosage.

Interactions:

Additive cholinergic effects. Do not use with depolarizing neuromuscular blocking agents. Use with ganglionic blocking agents may result in severe hypotension.

NURSING IMPLICATIONS

Assessment

- **General Info:** Monitor pulse, respiratory rate, and blood pressure frequently throughout parenteral administration.
- **Myasthenia Gravis:** Assess neuromuscular status (ptosis, diplopia, vital capacity, ability to swallow, and extremity strength) before and at time of peak effect.
- Assess patient for overdosage and underdosage or resistance. Both have similar symptoms (muscle weakness, dyspnea, and dysphagia), but symptoms of overdosage usually occur within 1 hr of administration, while underdosage symptoms occur 3 hr or more after administration. A Tensilon test (edrophonium chloride) may be used to distinguish between overdosage and underdosage.

---

*Because of space limitations, additional classes or drugs not represented in *Davis's Drug Guide for Nurses*, 7th edition, are provided in this *Pocket Companion*.

- **Antidote to Nondepolarizing Neuromuscular Blocking Agents:** Monitor reversal of effects of neuromuscular blocking agents with a peripheral nerve stimulator.
- **Urinary Retention:** Monitor intake and output ratios. Palpate abdomen for bladder distention. Catheterization may be done to assess postvoid residual.
- **Glaucoma:** Monitor patient for changes in vision, eye irritation, and persistent headache.
- **Toxicity and Overdose:** Atropine is the specific antidote.

Potential Nursing Diagnoses

- Urinary elimination, altered (Indications).
- Breathing pattern, ineffective (Indications).
- Knowledge deficit, related to medication regimen (Patient/Family Teaching).

Implementation

- **Myasthenia Gravis:** For patients who have difficulty chewing, medication may be administered 30 min before meals.

Patient/Family Teaching

- **General Info:** Instruct patients with myasthenia gravis to take medication exactly as ordered. Taking the dose late may result in myasthenic crisis. Taking the dose early may result in a cholinergic crisis. This regimen must be continued as a lifelong therapy.
- **Ophth:** Instruct patient on correct method of application of drops or ointment (see Appendix I).
- Explain to patient that pupil constriction and temporary stinging and blurring of vision are expected. Notify health care professional if blurred vision and brow ache persist.
- Caution patient that night vision may be impaired.
- Advise patient of the need for regular eye exams to monitor intraocular pressure and visual fields.

Evaluation

Effectiveness of therapy can be demonstrated by: ▪ Reversal of CNS symptoms secondary to anticholinergic excess resulting from drug overdosage or ingestion of poisonous plants ▪ Control of elevated intraocular pressure ▪ Increase in bladder function and tone ▪ Decrease in abdominal distention ▪ Relief of myasthenic symptoms ▪ Differentiation of myasthenic from cholinergic crisis ▪ Reversal of paralysis after anesthesia ▪ Resolution of supraventricular tachycardia.

Cholinergic Agents Included in *Davis's Drug Guide for Nurses*

cholinomimetic
bethanechol 102

cholinesterase inhibitors
demercarium 1161
echothiophate 1161

isoflurophate 1161
neostigmine 693
physostigmine 1161, 1179
pyridostigmine 860
tacrine 951

CORTICOSTEROIDS*

PHARMACOLOGIC PROFILE

General Use:

Used in replacement doses (20 mg of hydrocortisone or equivalent) to treat adrenocortical insufficiency. Larger doses are usually used for their anti-inflammatory, immunosuppressive, or antineoplastic activity. Used adjunctively in many other situations, including hypercalcemia and autoimmune diseases. Topical corticosteroids are used in a variety of inflammatory and allergic conditions. Inhalant corticosteroids are used in the chronic management of reversible airway disease (asthma); intranasal and ophthalmic corticosteroids are used in the management of chronic allergic and inflammatory conditions.

General Action and Information:

Produce profound and varied metabolic effects, in addition to modifying the normal immune response and suppressing inflammation. Available in a variety of dosage forms, including oral, injectable, topical, and inhalation. Prolonged used of large amounts of topical or inhaled agent may result in systemic absorption and/or adrenal suppression.

Contraindications:

Serious infections (except for certain forms of meningitis). Do not administer live vaccines to patients on larger doses.

Precautions:

Prolonged treatment will result in adrenal suppression. Do not discontinue abruptly. Additional doses may be needed during stress (surgery and infection). Safety in pregnancy and lactation not established. Long-term use in children will result in decreased growth. May mask signs of infection. Use lowest dose possible for shortest time possible. Alternate-day therapy is preferable during long-term treatment.

Interactions:

Additive hypokalemia with amphotericin B, potassium-losing diuretics, mezlocillin, piperacillin, and ticarcillin. Hypokalemia may increase the risk of cardiac glycoside toxicity. May increase requirements for insulin or oral hypoglycemic agents. Phenytoin, phenobarbital, and rifampin stimulate metabolism and may decrease effectiveness. Oral contraceptives may block metabolism. Cholestyramine and colestipol may decrease absorption.

NURSING IMPLICATIONS

Assessment

- These drugs are indicated for many conditions. Assess involved systems prior to and periodically throughout course of therapy.
- Assess patient for signs of adrenal insufficiency (hypotension, weight loss, weakness, nausea, vomiting, anorexia, lethargy, confusion, restlessness) prior to and periodically throughout course of therapy.
- Children should have periodic evaluations of growth.

---

*Because of space limitations, additional classes or drugs not represented in *Davis's Drug Guide for Nurses*, 7th edition, are provided in this *Pocket Companion*.

Potential Nursing Diagnoses

- Infection, risk for (Side Effects).
- Knowledge deficit, related to medication regimen (Patient/Family Teaching).
- Body image disturbance (Side Effects).

Implementation

- **General Info:** If dose is ordered daily or every other day, administer in the morning to coincide with the body's normal secretion of cortisol.
- **PO:** Administer with meals to minimize gastric irritation.

Patient/Family Teaching

- Emphasize need to take medication exactly as directed. Review symptoms of adrenal insufficiency that may occur when stopping the medication and that may be life-threatening.
- Encourage patients on long-term therapy to eat a diet high in protein, calcium, and potassium and low in sodium and carbohydrates.
- These drugs cause immunosuppression and may mask symptoms of infection. Instruct patient to avoid people with known contagious illnesses and to report possible infections. Advise patient to consult health care professional before receiving any vaccinations.
- Discuss possible effects on body image. Explore coping mechanisms.
- Advise patient to carry identification in the event of an emergency in which patient cannot relate medical history.

Evaluation

Effectiveness of therapy can be demonstrated by: ■ Suppression of the inflammatory and immune responses in autoimmune disorders, allergic reactions, and organ transplants ■ Replacement therapy in adrenal insufficiency ■ Resolution of skin inflammation, pruritus, or other dermatologic conditions.

Corticosteroids Included in *Davis's Drug Guide for Nurses*

corticosteroids, inhalation
beclomethasone 229
budesonide 229
flunisolide 229
fluticasone 229
triamcinolone 229

corticosteroids, nasal
beclomethasone 233
budesonide 233
dexamethasone 233
flunisolide 233

fluticasone 233
mometasone 233
triamcinolone 233

corticosteroids, ophthalmic
dexamethasone 1161
fluromethalone 1161
loteprednol 1161
medrysone 1161
prednisone 236
rimexolone 1161

*corticosteroids, systemic
(short-acting)*
cortisone 236
hydrocortisone 236

*corticosteroids, systemic
(intermediate-acting)*
methylprednisolone 236
prednisolone 236
prednisone 236
triamcinolone 236

*cocorticosteroids, systemic
(long-acting)*
betamethasone 236
dexamethasone 236

corticosteroids, topical/local
alclometasone 244
amcinonide 244

betamethasone 244
clobetasol 244
clocortolone 244
desonide 244
desoximetasone 244
dexamethasone 244
diflorasone 244
fluocinolone 244
fluocinonide 244
flurandrenolide 244
fluticasone 244
halcinonide 244
halobetasol 244
hydrocortisone 245
methylprednisolone 245
mometasone 245
prednicarbate 245
triamcinolone 245

DIURETICS

PHARMACOLOGIC PROFILE

General Use:

Thiazide and loop diuretics are used alone or in combination in the treatment of hypertension or edema due to congestive heart failure or other causes. Potassium-sparing diuretics have weak diuretic and antihypertensive properties and are used mainly to conserve potassium in patients receiving thiazide or loop diuretics. Osmotic diuretics are often used in the management of cerebral edema.

General Action and Information:

Enhance the selective excretion of various electrolytes and water by affecting renal mechanisms for tubular secretion and reabsorption. Groups commonly used are thiazide diuretics and thiazide-like diuretics (chlorothiazide, chlorthalidone, hydrochlorothiazide, indapamide, and metolazone), loop diuretics (bumetanide, furosemide, and toresemide), potassium-sparing diuretics (amiloride, spironolactone, and triamterene), and osmotic diuretics (mannitol). Mechanisms vary, depending on agent.

Contraindications:

Hypersensitivity. Thiazide diuretics may exhibit cross-sensitivity with other sulfonamides.

Precautions:

Use with caution in patients with renal or hepatic disease. Safety in pregnancy and lactation not established.

---

*Because of space limitations, additional classes or drugs not represented in *Davis's Drug Guide for Nurses*, 7th edition, are provided in this *Pocket Companion*.

Interactions:

Additive hypokalemia with corticosteroids, amphotericin B, mezlocillin, piperacillin, or ticarcillin. Hypokalemia enhances digitalis glycoside toxicity. Potassium-losing diuretics decrease lithium excretion and may cause toxicity. Additive hypotension with other antihypertensives or nitrates. Potassium-sparing diuretics may cause hyperkalemia when used with potassium supplements or ACE inhibitors.

NURSING IMPLICATIONS

Assessment

- **General Info:** Assess fluid status throughout therapy. Monitor daily weight, intake and output ratios, amount and location of edema, lung sounds, skin turgor, and mucous membranes.
- Assess patient for anorexia, muscle weakness, numbness, tingling, paresthesia, confusion, and excessive thirst. Notify physician or other health care professional promptly if these signs of electrolyte imbalance occur.
- **Hypertension:** Monitor blood pressure and pulse before and during administration. Monitor frequency of prescription refills to determine compliance in patients treated for hypertension.
- **Increased Intracranial Pressure:** Monitor neurologic status and intracranial pressure readings in patients receiving osmotic diuretics to decrease cerebral edema.
- **Increased Intraocular Pressure:** Monitor for persistent or increased eye pain or decreased visual acuity.
- **Lab Test Considerations:** Monitor electrolytes (especially potassium), blood glucose, BUN, and serum uric acid levels before and periodically throughout course of therapy.
- Thiazide diuretics may cause increased serum cholesterol, LDL, and triglyceride concentrations.

Potential Nursing Diagnoses

- Fluid volume excess (Indications).
- Knowledge deficit, related to medication regimen (Patient/Family Teaching).

Implementation

- Administer oral diuretics in the morning to prevent disruption of sleep cycle.
- Many diuretics are available in combination with antihypertensives or potassium-sparing diuretics.

Patient/Family Teaching

- **General Info:** Instruct patient to take medication exactly as directed. Advise patients on antihypertensive regimen to continue taking medication, even if feeling better. Medication controls but does not cure hypertension.
- Caution patient to make position changes slowly to minimize orthostatic hypotension. Caution patient that the use of alcohol, exercise during hot weather, or standing for long periods during therapy may enhance orthostatic hypotension.
- Instruct patient to consult health care professional regarding dietary potassium guidelines.
- Instruct patient to monitor weight weekly and report significant changes.
- Caution patient to use sunscreen and protective clothing to prevent photosensitivity reactions.
- Advise patient to consult health care professional before taking OTC medication concurrently with this therapy.

- Instruct patient to notify health care professional of medication regimen before treatment or surgery.
- Advise patient to contact health care professional immediately if muscle weakness, cramps, nausea, dizziness, or numbness or tingling of extremities occurs.
- Emphasize the importance of routine follow-up.
- **Hypertension:** Reinforce the need to continue additional therapies for hypertension (weight loss, regular exercise, restricted sodium intake, stress reduction, moderation of alcohol consumption, and cessation of smoking).
- Instruct patients with hypertension in the correct technique for monitoring weekly blood pressure.

Evaluation

Effectiveness of therapy can be demonstrated by: ■ Decreased blood pressure
n Increased urine output ■ Decreased edema ■ Reduced intracranial pressure ■ Prevention of hypokalemia in patients taking diuretics ■ Treatment of hyperaldosteronism.

Diuretics Included in *Davis's Drug Guide for Nurses*

loop diuretic
bumetanide 124
furosemide 315
toresemide 315

osmotic diuretic
mannitol 597

potassium-sparing diuretics
amiloride 312
spironolactone 312

triamterene 312

thiazide and thiazide-like diuretics
chlorothiazide 315
chlorthalidone 315
hydrochlorthiazide 315
indapamide 512
methyclothiazide 809
metolazone 636
trichlormethiazide 1176

ESTROGENS/PROGESTINS/HORMONAL CONTRACEPTIVES*

PHARMACOLOGIC PROFILE

General Use:

Used to treat hormonal deficiency states in menopausal women to minimize vasomotor symptoms and to prevent and treat osteoporosis. Estrogens and/or progestins are effective as oral contraceptives for women during the reproductive years.

General Action and Information:

Hormonal contraceptives block the ovulatory cycle through a negative feedback mechanism on the hypothalamus, by suppressing the production of follicle-stimulating hormone and luteinizing hormone. In addition to suppressing ovulation, these agents affect the movement of the ovum and sperm and creates an environment that is unfavorable for the implantation of a fertilized ovum. Estrogens promote the growth and development of female sex organs and the maintenance of secondary sex characteristics. Estrogens inhibit bone resorption in the prevention and treatment of osteoporosis.

---

*Because of space limitations, additional classes or drugs not represented in *Davis's Drug Guide for Nurses*, 7th edition, are provided in this *Pocket Companion*.

Contraindications:

Should not be used in thromboembolic disease, cerebrovascular accident or patients with a history of coronary artery or ischemic heart disease, pregnancy, breast cancer or patients with a history of breast cancer, and severe liver disease.

Precautions:

Use cautiously in women over age 35 who smoke heavily and in patients with hypertension, diabetes, renal disease, lactation, and family history of hyperlipidemia.

Interactions:

May alter requirement for warfarin, oral hypoglycemic agents, or insulin. Antibiotics and anticonvulsants (except valproic acid) may decrease effectiveness. Cigarette smoking increases the risk of adverse cardiovascular effects.

NURSING IMPLICATIONS

Assessment

- Assess blood pressure prior to the start of and periodically during therapy.
- Exclude thrombophlebitis and breast cancer by history or physical exam prior to initiating therapy.
- Exclude pregnancy prior to starting therapy.
- Assess smoking habits and encourage individuals to stop smoking while on hormonal therapy.
- Assess for history of gallbladder disease, hypertension, impaired liver function, obesity, and conditions that may be aggravated by fluid retention. Monitor these individuals at more frequent intervals.

Potential Nursing Diagnoses

- Noncompliance (Family/Patient Teaching).
- Knowledge deficit, related to medication regimen (Patient/Family Teaching).

Implementation

- Oral doses may be administered with or immediately after food to reduce nausea.
- Implant is inserted subdermally in midportion of upper arm about 8–10 cm above the elbow crease.
- Administer IM doses deep into the gluteal or deltoid muscle.

Patient/Family Teaching

- Instruct patient to take oral medication as directed at the same time each day. Pills should be taken in proper sequence and kept in the original container.
- Advise patient of need to use another form of contraception for the first 3 wk when beginning to use oral contraceptives.
- Warn patient that many other medications (e.g., certain antibiotics) may interfere with the action of oral contraceptives and to remind their health care professional that he or she is taking birth control pills whenever any other medications are prescribed for them.
- If nausea is a problem, advise patient that eating solid food often provides relief.

- Advise patient to report signs of fluid retention, thromboembolic disorders, mental depression, hepatic dysfunction, or abnormal vaginal bleeding.
- Inform patient to stop taking medication and to contact theirhealth care professional if pregnancy is suspected.
- Caution patient that cigarette smoking during estrogen therapy may increase the risk of serious side effects, especially for women over age 35.
- Warn patient to wear sunscreen and protective clothing to prevent increased pigmentation.
- Caution patient that oral contraceptives do not protect against HIV and other sexually transmitted diseases.
- Advise patient to notify health care professional of medication regimen prior to treatment or surgery.
- Emphasize the importance of routine follow-up exams, including blood pressure, breast, abdomen, pelvic, and PAP smears, every 6–12 mo.

Evaluation

Effectiveness of therapy can be demonstrated by: ■ Prevention of pregnancy ■ Regulation of menstrual cycle ■ Decrease in acne ■ Control of menopausal symptoms.

Estrogens/Progestins/Hormonal Contraceptives Included in *Davis's Drug Guide for Nurses*

estrogens
estrogens, conjugated 368
estropipate 371

progestins
medroxyprogesterone 605
progesterone 837

contraceptives, hormonal (monophasic)
ethinyl estradiol/desogestrel 225
ethinyl estradiol/ethynodiol 225
ethinyl estradiol/norethindrone 225
ethinyl estradiol/norgestrel 225

contraceptives, hormonal (biphasic)
ethinyl estradiol/northindrone 225

contraceptives, hormonal (triphasic)
ethinyl estradiol/norethindrone 225
ethinyl estradiol/norgestrel 225
ethinyl estradiol/norgestimate 225

progestin only
norethindrone 226
norgestrel 225

contraceptive implant
levonorgestrel 226

contraceptives, hormonal (emergency contraceptives)
ethinyl estradiol/levonorgestrel 225

IMMUNOSUPPRESSANT AGENTS*

PHARMACOLOGIC PROFILE

General Use:

Azathioprine, basiliximab, cyclosporine, daclizumab, mycophenolate, sirolimus, and tacrolimus are used with glucocorticoids in the prevention of transplantation rejection reactions. Muromonab-CD3 is used to manage rejection reactions not controlled by other agents. Azathioprine, cyclophosphamide, and methotrexate are used in the management of selected autoimmune diseases (nephrotic syndrome of childhood and severe rheumatoid arthritis).

---

*Because of space limitations, additional classes or drugs not represented in *Davis's Drug Guide for Nurses*, 7th edition, are provided in this *Pocket Companion*.

General Action and Information:

Inhibit cell-mediated immune responses by different mechanisms. In addition to azathioprine and cyclosporine, which are used primarily for their immunomodulating properties, cyclophosphamide and methotrexate are used to suppress the immune responses in certain disease states (nephrotic syndrome of childhood and severe rheumatoid arthritis). Muromonab-CD3 is a recombinant immunoglobulin antibody that alters T-cell function. Basiliximab and daclizumab are monoclonal antibodies.

Contraindications:

Hypersensitivity to drug or vehicle.

Precautions:

Use cautiously in patients with infections. Safety in pregnancy and lactation not established.

Interactions:

Allopurinol inhibits the metabolism of azathioprine. Drugs that alter liver-metabolizing processes may change the effect of cyclosporine. The risk to toxicity of methotrexate may be increased by other nephrotoxic drugs, large doses of aspirin, or NSAIDs. Muromonab-CD3 has additive immunosuppressive properties; concurrent immunosuppressive doses should be decreased or eliminated.

NURSING IMPLICATIONS

Assessment

- **General Info:** Monitor for infection (vital signs, sputum, urine, stool, WBC). Notify physician or other health care professional immediately if symptoms occur.
- **Organ Transplant:** Assess for symptoms of organ rejection throughout therapy.
- **Lab Test Considerations:** Monitor CBC and differential throughout therapy.

Potential Nursing Diagnoses

- Infection, risk for (Side Effects).
- Knowledge deficit, related to medication regimen (Patient/Family Teaching).

Implementation

- Protect transplant patients from staff and visitors who may carry infection.
- Maintain protective isolation as indicated.

Patient/Family Teaching

- Reinforce the need for lifelong therapy to prevent transplant rejection. Review symptoms of rejection for transplanted organ and stress need to notify health care professional immediately if they occur.
- Advise patient to avoid contact with contagious persons and those who have recently taken oral poliovirus vaccine. Patients should not receive vaccinations without first consulting with health care professional.
- Emphasize the importance of follow-up exams and lab tests.

Evaluation

Effectiveness of therapy can be demonstrated by: ■ Prevention or reversal of rejection of organ transplants or decrease in symptoms of autoimmune disorders.

Immunosuppressant Agents Included in *Davis's Drug Guide for Nurses*

azathioprine 85
basiliximab 92
cyclophosphamide 249
cyclosporine 252

methotrexate 627
muromonab-CD3 672
sirolimus 924

LAXATIVES

PHARMACOLOGIC PROFILE

General Use:

Used to treat or prevent constipation or to prepare the bowel for radiologic or endoscopic procedures.

General Action and Information:

Induce one or more bowel movements per day. Groups include stimulants (bisacodyl, senna), saline laxatives (magnesium salts and phosphates), stool softeners (docusate), bulk-forming agents (polycarbophil and psyllium), and osmotic cathartics (lactulose, polyethylene glycol/electrolyte). Increasing fluid intake, exercising, and adding more dietary fiber are also useful in the management of chronic constipation.

Contraindications:

Hypersensitivity. Contraindicated in persistent abdominal pain, nausea, or vomiting of unknown cause, especially if accompanied by fever or other signs of an acute abdomen.

Precautions:

Excessive or prolonged use may lead to dependence. Should not be used in children unless advised by a physician or other health care professional.

Interactions:

Theoretically may decrease the absorption of other orally administered drugs by decreasing transit time.

NURSING IMPLICATIONS

Assessment

- Assess patient for abdominal distention, presence of bowel sounds, and usual pattern of bowel function.
- Assess color, consistency, and amount of stool produced.

---

*Because of space limitations, additional classes or drugs not represented in *Davis's Drug Guide for Nurses*, 7th edition, are provided in this *Pocket Companion*.

Potential Nursing Diagnoses

■ Constipation (Indications).
■ Knowledge deficit, related to medication regimen (Patient/Family Teaching).

Implementation

■ Many laxatives may be administered at bedtime for morning results.
■ Taking oral doses on an empty stomach will usually produce more rapid results.
■ Do not crush or chew enteric-coated tablets. Take with a full glass of water or juice.
■ Stool softeners and bulk laxatives may take several days for results.

Patient/Family Teaching

■ Advise patients, other than those with spinal cord injuries, that laxatives should be used only for short-term therapy. Long-term therapy may cause electrolyte imbalance and dependence.
■ Advise patient to increase fluid intake to a minimum of 1500–2000 ml/day during therapy to prevent dehydration.
■ Encourage patients to use other forms of bowel regulation: increasing bulk in the diet, increasing fluid intake, and increasing mobility. Normal bowel habits are individualized and may vary from 3 times/day to 3 times/wk.
■ Instruct patients with cardiac disease to avoid straining during bowel movements (Valsalva maneuver).
■ Advise patient that laxatives should not be used when constipation is accompanied by abdominal pain, fever, nausea, or vomiting.

Evaluation

Effectiveness of therapy can be demonstrated by: ■ A soft, formed bowel movement ■ Evacuation of colon.

Laxatives Included in *Davis's Drug Guide for Nurses*

bulk-forming agents
polycarbophil 811
psyllium 858

osmotic agents
lactulose 557
polyethylene glycol/electrolyte 813

saline laxatives
magnesium citrate 593

magnesium hydroxide 593
phosphate/biphosphate 794

stimulants
bisacodyl 108
senna, sennosides 915

stool softener
docusate 322

LIPID-LOWERING AGENTS

PHARMACOLOGIC PROFILE

General Use:

Used as a part of a total plan including diet and exercise to reduce blood lipids in an effort to reduce the morbidity and mortality of atherosclerotic cardiovascular disease and its sequelae.

General Action and Information:

HMG-CoA reductase inhibitors (fluvastatin, lovastatin, pravastatin, simvastatin) inhibit an enzyme involved in cholesterol synthesis. Bile acid sequestrants (cholestyramine, colestipol) bind cholesterol in the GI tract. Niacin and gemfibrozil act by other mechanisms (see individual monographs).

Contraindications:

Hypersensitivity.

Precautions:

Safety in pregnancy, lactation, and children not established. See individual drugs. Dietary therapy should be given a 2–3 mo trial before drug therapy is initiated.

Interactions:

Bile acid sequestrants (cholestyramine and colestipol) may bind lipid-soluble vitamins (A, D, E, and K) and other concurrently administered drugs in the GI tract. The risk of myopathy from HMG-CoA reductase inhibitors is increased by niacin, erythromycin, gemfibrozil, and cyclosporine.

NURSING IMPLICATIONS

Assessment

- Obtain a diet history, especially in regard to fat and alcohol consumption.
- **Lab Test Considerations:** Serum cholesterol and triglyceride levels should be evaluated before initiating and periodically throughout therapy. Medication should be discontinued if paradoxical increase in cholesterol level occurs.
- Liver function tests should be assessed before and periodically throughout therapy. May cause an increase in levels.

Potential Nursing Diagnoses

- Knowledge deficit, related to medication regimen (Patient/Family Teaching).
- Noncompliance (Patient/Family Teaching).

Implementation

- See specific medications to determine timing of doses in relation to meals.

Patient/Family Teaching

- Advise patient that these medications should be used in conjunction with diet restrictions (fat, cholesterol, carbohydrates, and alcohol), exercise, and cessation of smoking.

Evaluation

Effectiveness of therapy can be demonstrated by: ■ Decreased serum triglyceride and LDL cholesterol levels and improved high-density lipoprotein HDL cholesterol ratios. Therapy is usually discontinued if the clinical response is not evident after 3 mo of therapy.

---

*Because of space limitations, additional classes or drugs not represented in *Davis's Drug Guide for Nurses*, 7th edition, are provided in this *Pocket Companion*.

Lipid-Lowering Agents Included in *Davis's Drug Guide for Nurses*

bile acid sequestrants
cholestyramine 105
colestipol 105

HMG-CoA reductase inhibitors
atorvastatin 478
cerivastatin 478
fluvastatin 478

lovastatin 478
pravastatin 478
simvastatin 478

miscellaneous
gemfibrozil 440
niacin, niacinamide 697

MINERALS/ELECTROLYTES*

PHARMACOLOGIC PROFILE

General Use:

Electrolytes are used to prevent or treat fluid and electrolyte imbalances and to maintain acid-base balance and osmotic pressure. Minerals are used to prevent or treat deficiencies in trace minerals.

General Action and Information:

Electrolytes are essential for homeostasis in the body. Maintenance of electrolyte levels within normal limits is necessary for many physiologic processes, such as cardiac, nerve, and muscle function, bone growth and stability; and others. Minerals are needed for normal growth and function; as cofactors in enzymatic reactions; and as stabilizing factors in hemoglobin synthesis, protein synthesis, and many other physiologic processes.

Contraindications:

Contraindicated in situations in which replacement would cause excess or when risk factors for fluid retention are present.

Precautions:

Use cautiously in disease states in which electrolyte imbalances are common, such as hepatic or renal disease, adrenal disorders, pituitary disorders, and diabetes mellitus.

Interactions:

See individual agents.

NURSING IMPLICATIONS

Assessment

- Observe patient carefully for evidence of electrolyte excess or insufficiency. Monitor lab values before and periodically throughout therapy.
- Nutrition, altered: less than body requirements (Indications).
- Knowledge deficit, related to medication and dietary regimens (Patient/Family Teaching).

Implementation

- **Potassium Chloride:** Do not administer parenteral potassium chloride undiluted.

Patient/Family Teaching

■ Review diet modifications with patients with chronic electrolyte disturbances.

Evaluation

Effectiveness of therapy can be demonstrated by: ■ Return to normal serum electrolyte concentrations and resolution of clinical symptoms of electrolyte imbalance ■ Changes in pH or composition of urine, which prevent formation of renal calculi.

Minerals/Electrolytes Included in *Davis's Drug Guide for Nurses*

calcium supplements
calcium acetate 142
calcium carbonate 142
calcium chloride 142
calcium citrate 142
calcium glubionate 142
calcium gluceptate 142
calcium gluconate 142
calcium lactate 142
tricalcium phosphate 142

iron supplements
carbonyl iron 532
ferrous fumarate 533
ferrous gluconate 533
ferrous sulfate 533
iron dextran 533
iron polysaccharide 533
sodium ferric gluconate complex 533

magnesium salts
magnesium salts (oral) 593

phosphate supplements
potassium phosphate 817
potassium and sodium phosphates 815
sodium phosphate 932

potassium supplements
potassium acetate 819
potassium bicarbonate 819
potassium chloride, 819
potassium citrate 819
potassium gluconate 820
trikates 820

miscellaneous
sodium bicarbonate 926
sodium chloride 928

NON-OPIOID ANALGESICS*

PHARMACOLOGIC PROFILE

General Use:

Used to control mild to moderate pain and/or fever. Phenazopyridine is used only to treat urinary tract pain, and capsaicin is used topically for a variety of painful syndromes.

General Action and Information:

Most non-opioid analgesics inhibit prostaglandin synthesis peripherally for analgesic effect and centrally for antipyretic effect.

Contraindications:

Hypersensitivity and cross-sensitivity among NSAIDs may occur.

Precautions:

Use cautiously in patients with severe hepatic or renal disease, chronic alcohol use/abuse, or malnutrition. Tramadol has CNS depressant properties.

---

*Because of space limitations, additional classes or drugs not represented in *Davis's Drug Guide for Nurses*, 7th edition, are provided in this *Pocket Companion*.

Interactions:

Chronic use of acetaminophen with NSAIDs may increase the risk of adverse renal effects. Chronic high-dose acetaminophen may increase the risk of bleeding with warfarin. Hepatotoxicity may be additive with other hepatotoxic agents, including alcohol. NSAIDs increase the risk of bleeding with warfarin, thrombolytic agents, antiplatelet agents, some cephalosporins, and valproates (effect is greatest with aspirin). NSAIDs may also decrease the effectiveness of diuretics and antihypertensives. The risk of CNS depression with tramadol is increased by concurrent use of other CNS depressants, including alcohol, antihistamines, sedative/hypnotics, and some antidepressants.

NURSING IMPLICATIONS

Assessment

- **General Info:** Patients who have asthma, allergies, and nasal polyps or who are allergic to tartrazine are at an increased risk for developing hypersensitivity reactions.
- **Pain:** Assess pain and limitation of movement; note type, location, and intensity prior to and at the peak (see Time/Action Profile) following administration.
- **Fever:** Assess fever and note associated signs (diaphoresis, tachycardia, malaise, chills).
- **Lab Test Considerations:** Hepatic, hematologic, and renal function should be evaluated periodically throughout prolonged, high-dose therapy. Aspirin and most NSAIDs prolong bleeding time due to suppressed platelet aggregation and, in large doses, may cause prolonged prothrombin time. Monitor hematocrit periodically in prolonged high-dose therapy to assess for GI blood loss.

Potential Nursing Diagnoses

- Pain (Indications).
- Body temperature, altered (Indications).
- Knowledge deficit related to medication regimen (Patient/Family Teaching).

Implementation

- **PO:** Administer salicylates and NSAIDs after meals or with food or an antacid to minimize gastric irritation.

Patient/Family Teaching

- Instruct patient to take salicylates and NSAIDs with a full glass of water and to remain in an upright position for 15–30 min after administration.
- Adults should not take acetaminophen longer than 10 days and children not longer than 5 days unless directed by health care professional. Short-term doses of acetaminophen with salicylates or NSAIDs should not exceed the recommended daily dose of either drug alone.
- Caution patient to avoid concurrent use of alcohol with this medication to minimize possible gastric irritation; 3 or more glasses of alcohol per day may increase the risk of GI bleeding with salicylates or NSAIDs. Caution patient to avoid taking acetaminophen, salicylates, or NSAIDs concurrently for more than a few days, unless directed by health care professional to prevent analgesic nephropathy.
- Advise patients on long-term therapy to inform health care professional of medication regimen prior to surgery. Aspirin, salicylates, and NSAIDs may need to be withheld prior to surgery.

Evaluation

Effectiveness of therapy can be demonstrated by: ■ Relief of mild to moderate discomfort ■ Reduction of fever.

Non-opioid Analgesics Included in *Davis's Drug Guide for Nurses*

nonsteroidal anti-inflammatory drugs
etodolac 379
ibuprofen 499
ketorolac 552
naproxen P–98

salicylates
aspirin 903

choline and magnesium salicylates 903
choline salicylate 903
salsalate 903

miscellaneous
acetaminophen 3
phenazopyridine 783
tramadol 1011

NONSTEROIDAL ANTI-INFLAMMATORY AGENTS*

PHARMACOLOGIC PROFILE

General Use:

NSAIDs are used to control mild to moderate pain, fever, and various inflammatory conditions, such as rheumatoid arthritis and osteoarthritis. Ophthalmic NSAIDs are used to decrease postoperative ocular inflammation, to inhibit perioperative miosis, and to decrease inflammation due to allergies.

General Action and Information:

NSAIDs have analgesic, antipyretic, and anti-inflammatory properties. Analgesic and anti-inflammatory effects are due to inhibition of prostaglandin synthesis. Antipyretic action is due to vasodilation and inhibition of prostaglandin synthesis in the CNS.

Contraindications:

Hypersensitivity to aspirin is a contraindication for the whole group of NSAIDs. Cross-sensitivity may occur.

Precautions:

Use cautiously in patients with a history of bleeding disorders, GI bleeding, and severe hepatic, renal, or cardiovascular disease. Safe use in pregnancy is not established and, in general, should be avoided during the second half of pregnancy.

Interactions:

NSAIDs prolong bleeding time and potentiate the effect of warfarin, thrombolytic agents, plicamycin, some cephalosporins, antiplatelet agents, and valproates. Chronic use with aspirin may result in increased GI side effects and decreased effectiveness. NSAIDs may also decrease response to diuretics or antihypertensive therapy.

---

*Because of space limitations, additional classes or drugs not represented in *Davis's Drug Guide for Nurses*, 7th edition, are provided in this *Pocket Companion*.

NURSING IMPLICATIONS

Assessment

- **General Info:** Patients who have asthma, allergies, and nasal polyps or who are allergic to tartrazine are at an increased risk for developing hypersensitivity reactions.
- **Pain:** Assess pain and limitation of movement; note type, location, and intensity prior to and at the peak (see Time/Action Profile) following administration.
- **Fever:** Assess fever and note associated signs (diaphoresis, tachycardia, malaise, chills).
- **Lab Test Considerations:** Most NSAIDs prolong bleeding time due to suppressed platelet aggregation and, in large doses, may cause prolonged prothrombin time. Monitor periodically in prolonged high-dose therapy to assess for GI blood loss.

Potential Nursing Diagnoses

- Pain (Indications).
- Body temperature, altered (Indications).
- Knowledge deficit, related to medication regimen (Patient/Family Teaching).

Implementation

- PO: Administer NSAIDs after meals or with food or an antacid to minimize gastric irritation.

Patient/Family Teaching

- Instruct patient to take NSAIDs with a full glass of water and to remain in an upright position for 15–30 min after administration.
- Caution patient to avaoid concurrent use of alcohol with this medication to minimize possible gastric irritation; 3 or more glasses of alcohol per day may increase the risk of GI bleeding with salicylates or NSAIDs. Caution patient to avoid taking acetaminophen, salicylates, or NSAIDs concurrently for more than a few days, unless directed by health care professional to prevent analgesic nephropathy.
- Advise patient on long-term therapy to inform health care professional of medication regimen prior to surgery. NSAIDs may need to be withheld prior to surgery.

Evaluation

Effectiveness of therapy can be demonstrated by: ■ Relief of mild to moderate discomfort. ■ Reduction of fever.

Nonsteroidal Anti-inflammatory Agents Included in *Davis's Drug Guide for Nurses*

nonsteroidal anti-inflammatory drugs
aspirin 903
celecoxib 166
choline and magnesium salicylates 903
choline salicylate 903
diclofenac 282
etodolac 378
flurbiprofen 423
ibuprofen 499

ketoprofen 550
ketorolac 522
nabumetone 677
naproxen P–98
oxaprozin 733
piroxicam 807
rofecoxib 898
salsalate 903
sulindac 946
tolmetin 1003

ophthalmic NSAIDs
diclofenac 1164
flurbiprofen 1164

ketorolac 1164
suprofen 1164

OPIOID ANALGESICS*

PHARMACOLOGIC PROFILE

General Use:

Management of moderate to severe pain. Fentanyl is used as a general anesthetic adjunct.

General Action and Information:

Opioids bind to opiate receptors in the CNS, where they act as agonists of endogenously occurring opioid peptides (eukephalins and endorphins). The result is alteration to the perception of and response to pain.

Contraindications:

Hypersensitivity to individual agents.

Precautions:

Use cautiously in patients with undiagnosed abdominal pain, head trauma or pathology, liver disease, or history of addiction to opioids. Use smaller doses initially in the elderly and those with respiratory diseases. Chronic use may result in tolerance and the need for larger doses to relieve pain. Psychological or physical dependence may occur.

Interactions:

Increases the CNS depressant properties of other drugs, including alcohol, antihistamines, antidepressants, sedative/hypnotics, phenothiazines, and MAO inhibitors. Use of partial-antagonist opioid analgesics (buprenorphine, butorphanol, dezocine, nalbuphine, and pentazocine) may precipitate opioid withdrawal in physically dependent patients. Use with MAO inhibitors or procarbazine may result in severe paradoxical reactions (especially with meperidine). Nalbuphine or pentazocine may decrease the analgesic effects of other concurrently administered opioid analgesics.

NURSING IMPLICATIONS

Assessment

- Assess type, location, and intensity of pain prior to and at peak following administration. When titrating opioid doses, increases of 25–50% should be administered until there is either a 50% reduction in the patient's pain rating on a numerical or visual analogue scale or the patient reports satisfactory pain relief. A repeat dose can be safely administered at the time of the peak if previous dose is ineffective and side effects are minimal. Patients requiring higher doses of opioid agonist-antagonists should be converted to an opioid agonist. Opioid agonist-antagonists are not recommended for prolonged use or as first-line therapy for acute or cancer pain.
- An equianalgesic chart (see Appendix C) should be used when changing routes or when changing from one opioid to another.

---

*Because of space limitations, additional classes or drugs not represented in *Davis's Drug Guide for Nurses*, 7th edition, are provided in this *Pocket Companion*.

- Assess blood pressure, pulse, and respirations before and periodically during administration. If respiratory rate is <10/min, assess level of sedation. Physical stimulation may be sufficient to prevent significant hypoventilation. Dose may need to be decreased by 25–50%. Initial drowsiness will diminish with continued use.
- Assess prior analgesic history. Antagonistic properties of agonist-antagonists may induce withdrawal symptoms (vomiting, restlessness, abdominal cramps, and increased blood pressure and temperature) in patients physically dependent on opioids.
- Prolonged use may lead to physical and psychological dependence and tolerance. This should not prevent patient from receiving adequate analgesia. Most patients who receive opioid analgesics for pain do not develop psychological dependence. Progressively higher doses may be required to relieve pain with long-term therapy.
- Assess bowel function routinely. Prevention of constipation should be instituted with increased intake of fluids and bulk, stool softeners, and laxatives to minimize constipating effects. Stimulant laxatives should be administered routinely if opioid use exceeds 2–3 days, unless contraindicated.
- Monitor intake and output ratios. If significant discrepancies occur, assess for urinary retention and inform physician or other health care professional.
- **Toxicity and Overdose:** If an opioid antagonist is required to reverse respiratory depression or coma, naloxone (Narcan) is the antidote. Dilute the 0.4-mg ampule of naloxone in 10 ml of 0.9% NaCl and administer 0.5 ml (0.02 mg) by direct IV push every 2 min. For children and patients weighing <40 kg, dilute 0.1 mg of naloxone in 10 ml of 0.9% NaCl for a concentration of 10 mcg/ml and administer 0.5 mcg/kg every 1–2 min. Titrate dose to avoid withdrawal, seizures, and severe pain.

Potential Nursing Diagnoses

- Pain (Indications).
- Sensory-perceptual alteration: visual, auditory (Side Effects).
- Injury, risk for (Side Effects).
- Knowledge deficit, related to medication regimen (Patient/Family Teaching).

Implementation

- Do not confuse morphine with hydromorphone or meperidine; errors have resulted in fatalities.
- Explain therapeutic value of medication before administration to enhance the analgesic effect.
- Regularly administered doses may be more effective than prn administration. Analgesic is more effective if given before pain becomes severe.
- Coadministration with nonopioid analgesics may have additive analgesic effects and may permit lower doses.
- Medication should be discontinued gradually after long-term use to prevent withdrawal symptoms.

Patient/Family Teaching

- Instruct patient on how and when to ask for pain medication.
- Medication may cause drowsiness or dizziness. Caution patient to call for assistance when ambulating or smoking and to avoid driving or other activities requiring alertness until response to medication is known.
- Advise patient to make position changes slowly to minimize orthostatic hypotension.
- Caution patient to avoid concurrent use of alcohol or other CNS depressants with this medication.

- Encourage patient to turn, cough, and breathe deeply every 2 hr to prevent atelectasis.

Evaluation

Effectiveness of therapy can be demonstrated by: ■ Decreased severity of pain without a significant alteration in level of consciousness or respiratory status.

Opioid Analgesics Included in *Davis's Drug Guide for Nurses*

opioid agonists
codeine 221
fentanyl (parenteral) 391
fentanyl (transdermal) 394
fentanyl (transmucosal) 1176
hydrocodone 482
hydromorphone 486
meperidine 611
methadone 621
morphine 666

oxycodone, P-101
oxymorphone 1119
propoxyphene 847

opioid agonists/antagonists
buprenorphine 127
butorphanol 137
dezocine 1120
pentazocine 724

SKELETAL MUSCLE RELAXANTS

PHARMACOLOGIC PROFILE

General Use:

Two major uses are spasticity associated with spinal cord diseases or lesions (baclofen and dantrolene) or adjunctive therapy in the symptomatic relief of acute painful musculoskeletal conditions (cyclobenzaprine, diazepam, and methocarbamol). IV dantrolene is also used to treat and prevent malignant hyperthermia.

General Action and Information:

Act either centrally (baclofen, carisoprodol, cyclobenzaprine, diazepam, and methocarbamol) or directly (dantrolene).

Contraindications:

Baclofen and oral dantrolene should not be used in patients in whom spasticity is used to maintain posture and balance.

Precautions:

Safety in pregnancy and lactation not established. Use cautiously in patients with a previous history of liver disease.

Interactions:

Additive CNS depression with other CNS depressants, including alcohol, antihistamines, antidepressants, opioid analgesics, and sedative/hypnotics.

---

*Because of space limitations, additional classes or drugs not represented in *Davis's Drug Guide for Nurses*, 7th edition, are provided in this *Pocket Companion*.

NURSING IMPLICATIONS

Assessment

- Assess patient for pain, muscle stiffness, and range of motion before and periodically throughout therapy.

Potential Nursing Diagnoses

- Pain (Indications).
- Physical mobility, impaired (Indications).
- Injury, risk for (Side Effects).

Implementation

- Provide safety measures as indicated. Supervise ambulation and transfer of patients.

Patient/Family Teaching

- Encourage patient to comply with additional therapies prescribed for muscle spasm (rest, physical therapy, heat).
- Medication may cause drowsiness. Caution patient to avoid driving or other activities requiring alertness until response to drug is known.
- Advise patient to avoid concurrent use of alcohol or other CNS depressants with these medications.

Evaluation

Effectiveness of therapy can be demonstrated by: ■ Decreased musculoskeletal pain ■ Decreased muscle spasticity ■ Increased range of motion ■ Prevention or decrease in temperature and skeletal rigidity in malignant hyperthermia.

Skeletal Muscle Relaxants Included in *Davis's Drug Guide for Nurses*

centrally acting
baclofen 91
carisoprodol 157
chlorzoxazone 195
cyclobenzaprine 247
diazepam 279

methocarbamol 626
orphenadrine 1178

direct-acting
dantrolene 262

THROMBOLYTIC AGENTS*

PHARMACOLOGIC PROFILE

General Use:

Acute management of coronary thrombosis (myocardial infarction). Streptokinase and urokinase are used in the management of massive pulmonary emboli, deep vein thrombosis, and arterial thromboembolism. Alteplase is used in the management of acute ischemic stroke.

General Action and Information:

Converts plasminogen to plasmin, which then degrades fibrin in clots. Alteplase, reteplase, and urokinase directly activate plasminogen. Anistreplase and streptokinase bind with plasminogen to form activator complexes, which then convert plasminogen to plasmin. Results in lysis of thrombi in coronary arteries, pulmonary emboli, or deep vein thrombosis, or clearing of clots in cannulae/catheters.

Contraindications:

Hypersensitivity. Cross-sensitivity with anistreplase and streptokinase may occur. Contraindicated in active internal bleeding, history of cerebrovascular accident, recent CNS trauma or surgery, neoplasm, or arteriovenous malformation. Severe uncontrolled hypertension and known bleeding tendencies.

Precautions:

Recent (within 10 days) major surgery, trauma, GI or GU bleeding. Severe hepatic or renal disease. Subacute bacterial endocarditis or acute pericarditis. Use cautiously in geriatric patients. Safety not established in pregnancy, lactation, or children.

Interactions:

Concurrent use with aspirin, NSAIDs, warfarin, heparins, abciximab, ticlopidine, or dipyridamole may increase the risk of bleeding, although these agents are frequently used together or in sequence. Risk of bleeding may also be increased by concurrent use with cefamandole, cefotetan, cefoperazone, plicamycin, and valproic acid.

NURSING IMPLICATIONS

Assessment

- Begin therapy as soon as possible after the onset of symptoms.
- Monitor vital signs, including temperature, continuously for coronary thrombosis and at least every 4 hr during therapy for other indications. Do not use lower extremities to monitor blood pressure.
- Assess patient carefully for bleeding every 15 min during the 1st hr of therapy, every 15–30 min during the next 8 hr, and at least every 4 hr for the duration of therapy. Frank bleeding may occur from sites of invasive procedures or from body orifices. Internal bleeding may also occur (decreased neurologic status; abdominal pain with coffee-ground emesis or black, tarry stools; hematuria; joint pain). If uncontrolled bleeding occurs, stop medication and notify physician immediately.
- Inquire about previous reaction to anistreplase or streptokinase therapy. Assess patient for hypersensitivity reaction (rash, dyspnea, fever, changes in facial color, swelling around the eyes, wheezing). If these occur, inform physician promptly. Keep epinephrine, an antihistamine, and resuscitation equipment close by in the event of an anaphylactic reaction.
- Inquire about recent streptococcal infection. Anistreplase and streptokinase may be less effective if administered between 5 days and 6 mo of a streptococcal infection.
- Assess neurologic status throughout therapy.
- Altered sensorium or neurologic changes may be indicative of intracranial bleeding.
- **Coronary Thrombosis:** Monitor ECG continuously. Notify physician if significant arrhythmias occur. IV lidocaine or procainamide (Pronestyl) may be ordered prophylactically. Cardiac

*Because of space limitations, additional classes or drugs not represented in *Davis's Drug Guide for Nurses*, 7th edition, are provided in this *Pocket Companion*.

enzymes should be monitored. Radionuclide myocardial scanning and/or coronary angiography may be ordered 7–10 days following therapy to monitor effectiveness of therapy.

- Monitor heart sounds and breath sounds frequently. Inform physician if signs of congestive heart failure occur (rales/crackles, dyspnea, S_3 heart sound, jugular venous distention, relieved CVP).
- Monitor heart sounds and breath sounds frequently. Inform physician if signs of congestive heart failure occur (rales/crackles, dyspnea, S_3 heart sound, jugular venous distention, relieved CVP).
- **Pulmonary Embolism:** Monitor pulse, blood pressure, hemodynamics, and respiratory status (rate, degree of dyspnea, ABGs).
- **Deep Vein Thrombosis/Acture Arterial Occlusion:** Observe extremities and palpate pulses of affected extremities every hour. Notify physician immediately if circulatory impairment occurs. Computerized axial tomography, impedance plethysmography, quantitative Doppler effect determination, and/or angiography or venography may be used to determine restoration of blood flow and duration of therapy; however, repeated venograms are not recommended.
- **Cannula/Catheter Occlusion:** Monitor ability to aspirate blood as indicator of patency. Ensure that patient exhales and holds breath when connecting and disconnecting IV syringe to prevent air embolism.
- **Acute Ischemic Stroke:** Assess neurologic status. Determine time of onset of stroke symptoms. Alteplase must be administered within 3 hr of onset.
- **Lab Test Considerations:** Hematocrit, hemoglobin, platelet count, fibrin/fibrindegradation product (FDP/fdp) titer, fibrinogen concentration, prothrombin time, thrombin time, and activated partial thromboplastin time may be evaluated prior to and frequently throughout therapy. Bleeding time may be assessed prior to therapy if patient has received platelet aggregation inhibitors. Obtain type and crossmatch and have blood available at all times in case of hemorrhage. Stools should be tested for occult blood loss and urine for hematuria periodically during therapy
- **Toxicity and Overdose:**If local bleeding occurs, apply pressure to site. If severe or internal bleeding occurs, discontinue infusion. Clotting factors and/or blood volume may be restored through infusions of whole blood, packed RBCs, fresh frozen plasma, or cryoprecipitate. Do not administer dextran, as it has antiplatelet activity. Aminocaproic acid (Amicar) may be used as an antidote.

Potential Nursing Diagnoses

- Tissue perfusion (Indications).
- Injury, risk for (Side effects).
- Knowledge deficit, related to medication regimen (Patient/Family Teaching).

Implementation

- This medication should be used only in settings in which hematologic
- function and clinical response can be adequately monitored.
- Starting two IV lines prior to therapy is recommended: one for the thrombolytic agent, the other for any additional infusions.
- Avoid invasive procedures, such as IM injections or arterial punctures,with this therapy. If such procedures must be performed, apply pressure to all arterial and venous puncture sites for at least 30 min. Avoid venipunctures at noncompressible sites (jugular vein, subclavian site).
- Systemic anticoagulation with heparin is usually begun several hours after the completion of thrombolytic therapy.
- Acetaminophen may be ordered to control fever.

Patient/Family Teaching

■ Explain purpose of medication and the need for close monitoring to patient and family. Instruct patient to report hypersensitivity reactions (rash, dyspnea) and bleeding or bruising.
■ Explain need for bedrest and minimal handling during therapy to avoid injury. Avoid all unnecessary procedures such as shaving and vigorous tooth brushing.

Evaluation

Effectiveness of therapy can be demonstrated by: ■ Lysis of thrombi and restoration of blood flow ■ Prevention of neurologic sequelae in acute ischemic stroke ■ Cannula or catheter patency.

Thrombolytic Agents Included in *Davis's Drug Guide for Nurses*

alteplase 980	streptokinase 980
anistreplase 980	urokinase 980
reteplase 980	

VASCULAR HEADACHE SUPPRESSANTS

PHARMACOLOGIC PROFILE

General Use:

Used for acute treatment of vascular headaches (migraine, cluster headaches, migraine variants). Other agents such as some beta-adrenergic blockers and some calcum channel blockers are used for suppression of frequently occurring vascular headaches.

General action and information:

Ergot derivative agents (ergotamine, dihydroergotamine) directly stimulate alpha-adrenergic and serotonergic receptors, producing vascular smooth muscle vasoconstriction. Sumatriptan and zolmitriptan produce vasoconstriction by acting as serotonin agonists.

Contraindications:

Avoid using these agents in patients with ischemic cardiovascular disease.

Precautions:

Use cautiously in patients with a history of or risk for cardiovascular disease.

Interactions:

Avoid concurrent use of ergot derivative agents with serotonin agonist agents; see also individual agents.

---

*Because of space limitations, additional classes or drugs not represented in *Davis's Drug Guide for Nurses*, 7th edition, are provided in this *Pocket Companion*.

NURSING IMPLICATIONS

Assessment

- Assess pain location, intensity, duration, and associated symptoms (photophobia, phonophobia, nausea, vomiting) during migraine attack.

Potential Nursing Diagnoses

- Pain (Indications).
- Knowledge deficit, related to medication regimen (Patient/Family Teaching).

Implementation

- Medication should be administered at the first sign of a headache.

Patient/Family Teaching

- Inform patient that medication should be used only during a migraine attack. It is meant to be used for relief of migraine attacks but not to prevent or reduce the number of attacks.
- Advise patient that lying down in a darkened room following medication administration may further help relieve headache.
- May cause dizziness or drowsiness. Caution patient to avoid driving or other activities requiring alertness until response to medication is known.
- Advise patient to avoid alcohol, which aggravates headaches.

Evaluation

Effectiveness of therapy can be demonstrated by: ■ Relief of migraine attack.

Vascular Headache Suppressants Included in *Davis's Drug Guide for Nurses*

ergot derivatives
dihydroergotamine 357
ergotamine 357
naratriptan 688
rizatriptan 896

serotonin agonists
sumatriptan 947
zolmitriptan 1070

VITAMINS

PHARMACOLOGIC PROFILE

General Use:

Used in the prevention and treatment of vitamin deficiencies and as supplements in various metabolic disorders.

General Action and Information:

Serve as components of enzyme systems that catalyze numerous varied metabolic reactions. Necessary for homeostasis. Water-soluble vitamins (B-vitamins and vitamin C) rarely cause toxicity. Fat-soluble vitamins (vitamins D and E) may accumulate and cause toxicity.

Contraindications:

Hypersensitivity to additives, preservatives, or colorants.

Precautions:

Dosage should be adjusted to avoid toxicity, especially for fat-soluble vitamins.

Interactions:

Pyridoxine in large amounts may interfere with the effectiveness of levodopa. Cholestyramine, colestipol, and mineral oil decrease absorption of fat-soluble vitamins.

NURSING IMPLICATIONS

Assessment

- Assess patient for signs of vitamin deficiency before and periodically throughout therapy.
- Assess nutritional status through 24-hr diet recall. Determine frequency of consumption of vitamin-rich foods.

Potential Nursing Diagnoses

- Nutrition, altered: less than body requirements (Indications).
- Knowledge deficit, related to medication regimen (Patient/Family Teaching).

Implementation

- Because of infrequency of single vitamin deficiencies, combinations are commonly administered.

Patient/Family Teaching

- Encourage patients to comply with diet recommendations of physician or other health care professional. Explain that the best source of vitamins is a well-balanced diet with foods from the four basic food groups.
- Patients self-medicating with vitamin supplements should be cautioned not to exceed RDA (see Appendix M). The effectiveness of megadoses for treatment of various medical conditions is unproved and may cause side effects and toxicity.

Evaluation

Effectiveness of therapy may be demonstrated by: ■ Prevention of or decrease in the symptoms of vitamin deficiencies.

Vitamins Included in *Davis's Drug Guide for Nurses*

fat-soluble vitamins
calcitriol 1050
dihydrotachysterol 1050
ergocalciferol 1050
paricalcitol 1050
phytonadione (vitamin K) 795

vitamin D compounds 1050
vitamin E 1053

water-soluble vitamins
ascorbic acid (vitamin C) 75
cyanocobalamin (vitamin B_{12}) 1047
folic acid 428

---

*Because of space limitations, additional classes or drugs not represented in *Davis's Drug Guide for Nurses*, 7th edition, are provided in this *Pocket Companion*.

hydroxocobalamin (vitamin B$_{12}$) 1048
niacin, niacinamide (vitamin B$_3$) 697
pyridoxine (vitamin B$_6$) 863

riboflavin (vitamin B$_2$) 883
thiamine (vitamin B$_1$) 974

SECTION II

Drugs Not Represented in
Davis's Drug Guide for Nurses, 7th Edition*

CALCITONIN (human)
(kal-si-**toe**-nin)
Cibacalcin

CALCITONIN (salmon)
Calcimar, Miacalcin, Osteocalcin, Salmonine

CLASSIFICATION(S):
Calcium/phosphorous regulating hormones (hypocalcemic)

Pregnancy Category C

INDICATIONS

■ **IM, SC:** Treatment of Paget's disease of bone ■ Adjunctive therapy for hypercalcemia ■ **IM, SC, Intranasal:** Management of postmenopausal osteoporosis.

ACTION

■ Decreases serum calcium by a direct effect on bone, kidney, and GI tract ■ Promotes renal excretion of calcium. **Therapeutic Effects:** ■ Decreased rate of bone turnover ■ Lowering of serum calcium.

PHARMACOKINETICS

Absorption: Completely absorbed from IM and SC sites. Rapidly absorbed from nasal mucosa; absorption is 3% compared with parenteral administration.

Distribution: Unknown.

Metabolism and Excretion: Rapidly metabolized in kidneys, blood, and tissues.

Half-life: 70–90 min.

CONTRAINDICATIONS AND PRECAUTIONS

Contraindicated in: ■ Hypersensitivity to salmon protein or gelatin diluent ■ Pregnancy or lactation (use not recommended).

Use Cautiously in: ■ Children (safety not established).

ADVERSE REACTIONS AND SIDE EFFECTS†

CNS: headaches.
EENT: *nasal only*—epistaxis, nasal irritation, rhinitis.
GI: *IM, SC*—nausea, vomiting, altered taste, diarrhea.
GU: *IM, SC*—urinary frequency.
Derm: rashes.
Local: injection site reactions.
MS: *nasal*—arthralgia, back pain.
Misc: allergic reactions including ANAPHYLAXIS, facial flushing, swelling, tingling, and tenderness in the hands.

INTERACTIONS

Drug-Drug: ■ Previous bisphosphanate therapy, including **alendronate**, **etidronate** and **pamidronate** may decrease response to calcitonin.

ROUTE AND DOSAGE

❑ **Postmenopausal osteoporosis**
■ **IM, SC (Adults):** 100 IU/day.
■ **Intranasal (Adults):** 200 IU/day.

❑ **Paget's disease**
■ **IM, SC (Adults):** 100 IU/day initially, after titration, maintenance dose is usually 50IU/day or every other day.

*Because of space limitations, additional classes or drugs not represented in *Davis's Drug Guide for Nurses*, 7th edition, are provided in this *Pocket Companion*.

{ } = Available in Canada only.

†CAPITALS indicate life-threatening; underlines indicate most frequent.

□ Hypercalcemia

■ **IM, SC (Adults):** 4 IU/kg q 12 hr; may be increased after 1–2 days to 8 IU/kg q 12 hr, and if necessary after 2 more days may be increased to 8 IU q 6 hr.

AVAILABILITY

■ **Injection :** 200 IU/ml in 2 ml vials[Rx] ■ Cost: $34.00-53.40/vial ■ **Nasal spray:** 200 IU/ actuation in 2 ml bottles [Rx] ■ Cost:$56.72/bottle.

TIME/ACTION PROFILE

	ONSET	PEAK	DURATION
IM, SC*	Unknown	2 hr	6–8 hr
Intranasal[†]	rapid	31–39 min	Unknown

*Effects on serum calcium.
[†]Serum levels of administered calcitonin.

NURSING IMPLICATIONS

ASSESSMENT

□ Observe patient for signs of hypersensitivity (skin rash, fever, hives, anaphylaxis, serum sickness). Keep epinephrine, antihistamines, and oxygen nearby in the event of a reaction.

□ Assess patient for signs of hypocalcemic tetany (nervousness, irritability, paresthesia, muscle twitching, tetanic spasms, convulsions) during the first several doses of calcitonin. Parenteral calcium, such as calcium gluconate, should be available in case of this event.

■ *Lab Test Considerations:* Serum calcium and alkaline phosphatase should be monitored periodically throughout therapy. These levels should normalize within a few months of initiation of therapy.

□ Urine hydroxyproline (24 hr) may be monitored periodically in patients with Paget's disease.

POTENTIAL NURSING DIAGNOSES

■ Pain (Indications).

■ Injury, risk for (Indications, Side Effects).

■ Knowledge deficit, related to medication regimen (Patient/Family Teaching).

IMPLEMENTATION

■ **General Info:** Assess for sensitivity to calcitonin-salmon by administering an intradermal test dose on the inner aspect of the forearm prior to initiating therapy. Test dose is prepared in a dilution of 10 IU/ml by withdrawing 0.05 ml in a tuberculin syringe and filling to 1 ml with 0.9% NaCl for injection. Mix well and discard 0.9 ml. Administer 0.1 ml and observe site for 15 min. More than mild erythema or wheal constitutes positive response.

□ Store solution in refrigerator.

■ **IM, SC:** Inspect injection site for the appearance of redness, swelling, or pain. Rotate injection sites. SC is the preferred route. Use IM route if dose exceeds 2 ml in volume. Use multiple sites to minimize inflammatory reaction.

□ Do not administer solutions that are discolored or contain particulate matter.

PATIENT/FAMILY TEACHING

■ **General Info:** Advise patient to take medication exactly as directed. If dose is missed and medication is scheduled for twice a day, take only if possible within 2 hr of correct time. If scheduled for daily dose, take only if remembered that day. If scheduled for every other day, take when remembered and restart alternate day schedule. If taking 1 dose 3 times weekly (Mon, Wed, Fri), take missed dose the next day and set each injection back 1 day; resume regular schedule the following week. Do not double doses.

□ Instruct patient in the proper method of self-injection.

□ Advise patient to report signs of hypercalcemic relapse (deep bone or flank pain, renal calculi, anorexia, nausea, vomiting, thirst, lethargy) or allergic response promptly.

□ Reassure patient that flushing and warmth following injection are transient and usually last about 1 hr.

□ Explain that nausea following injection tends to decrease even with continued therapy.

□ Instruct patient to follow low-calcium diet if recommended by health care professional (see Appendix L). Women with postmenopausal osteoporosis should adhere to a diet high in calcium and vitamin D.

■ **Osteoporosis:** Advise patients receiving calcitonin for the treatment of osteoporosis that exercise has been found to arrest and reverse bone loss. The patient should discuss any exercise limitations with health care professional before beginning program.

■ **Intranasal:** Instruct patient on correct use of nasal spray. Before first use, activate pump by holding upright and depressing white side arms down toward bottle 6 times until a fine spray is emitted. Following activation, place nozzle firmly in nostril with head in an upright position and depress the pump toward the bottle.

❑ Advise patient to notify health care professional if significant nasal irritation occurs.

EVALUATION

Effectiveness of therapy can be demonstrated by: ■ Lowered serum calcium levels ■ Decreased bone pain ■ Slowed progression of postmenopausal osteoporosis. Significant increases in bone marrow density may be seen as early as a month after initiation of therapy.

FEXOFENADINE
(fex-oh-**fen**-a-deen)
Allegra

CLASSIFICATION(S):
Antihistamines

Pregnancy Category C

INDICATIONS

■ Relief of symptoms of seasonal allergic rhinitis.

ACTION

■ Antagonizes the effects of histamine at peripheral histamine-1 (H_1) receptors, including pruritus and urticaria ■ Also has a drying effect on the nasal mucosa. Therapeutic Effects: ■ Decreased sneezing, rhinorrhea, itchy eyes, nose, and throat associated with seasonal allergies.

PHARMACOKINETICS

Absorption: Rapidly absorbed after oral administration.
Distribution: Unknown.
Metabolism and Excretion: 80% excreted in urine, 11% excreted in feces.
Half-life: 14.4 hr (increased in renal impairment).

CONTRAINDICATIONS AND PRECAUTIONS

Contraindicated in: ■ Hypersensitivity.
Use Cautiously in: ■ Impaired renal function (increased dosing interval recommended) ■ Pregnancy, lactation, or children <12 yr (safety not established).

ADVERSE REACTIONS AND SIDE EFFECTS†

CNS: drowsiness, fatigue.
GI: dyspepsia.
Endo: dysmenorrhea.

INTERACTIONS

Drug-Drug: ■ None significant.

ROUTE AND DOSAGE

■ **PO (Adults and Children ≥12 yr):** 60 mg twice daily.

❑ **Renal Impairment**
■ **PO (Adults):** 60 mg once daily.

AVAILABILITY

■ *Capsules:* 60 mg^{Rx} ■Cost: $99.42/100 ■ *In combination with:* pseudoephedrine (Allegra-D^{Rx}). See Appendix B.

TIME/ACTION PROFILE (antihistaminic effect)

	ONSET	PEAK	DURATION
PO	within 1 hr	2–3 hr	12 hr

NURSING IMPLICATIONS

ASSESSMENT

❑ Assess allergy symptoms (rhinitis, conjunctivitis, hives) before and periodically throughout therapy.
❑ Assess lung sounds and character of bronchial secretions. Maintain fluid intake of 1500–2000 ml/day to decrease viscosity of secretions.
■ *Lab Test Considerations:* Will cause false-negative reactions on allergy skin tests; discontinue 3 days before testing.

POTENTIAL NURSING DIAGNOSES

- Ineffective airway clearance (Indications).
- Injury, risk for (Adverse Reactions).
- Knowledge deficit, related to medication regimen (Patient/Family Teaching).

IMPLEMENTATION

- **PO:** Administer with food or milk to decrease GI irritation.

PATIENT/FAMILY TEACHING

- ❏ Instruct patient to take medication as directed. If a dose is missed, take as soon as remembered unless almost time for next dose.
- ❏ Inform patient that drug may cause drowsiness, although it is less likely to occur than with other antihistamines. Avoid driving or other activities requiring alertness until response to drug is known.
- ❏ Instruct patient to contact health care professional if symptoms persist.

EVALUATION

Effectiveness of therapy can be demonstrated by: ■ Decrease in allergic symptoms.

METHYLDOPA
(meth-ill-**doe**-pa)
Aldomet, {Apo-Methyldopa},
{Dopamet}, {Novamedopa},
{Nu-Medopa}

CLASSIFICATION(S):
Antihypertensive agents (centrally acting alpha-adrenergic agonist)

Pregnancy Category B

INDICATIONS

- Management of moderate to severe hypertension (with other agents).

ACTION

- Stimulates CNS alpha-adrenergic receptors, producing a decrease in sympathetic outflow to heart, kidneys, and blood vessels. Result is decreased blood pressure and peripheral resistance, a slight decrease in heart rate, and no change in cardiac output. **Therapeutic Effects:** ■ Lowering of blood pressure.

PHARMACOKINETICS

Absorption: 50% absorbed from the GI tract. Parenteral form, methyldopate hydrochloride, is slowly converted to methyldopa.
Distribution: Crosses the blood-brain barrier. Crosses the placenta; small amounts enter breast milk.
Metabolism and Excretion: Partially metabolized by the liver, partially excreted unchanged by the kidneys.
Half-life: 1.7 hr.

CONTRAINDICATIONS AND PRECAUTIONS

Contraindicated in: ■ Hypersensitivity ■ Active liver disease ■ Some products contain alcohol or bisulfites and should be avoided in patients with known intolerance.
Use Cautiously in: ■ Previous history of liver disease ■ Geriatric patients (increased risk of adverse reactions) ■ Pregnancy (has been used safely) ■ Lactation.

ADVERSE REACTIONS AND SIDE EFFECTS†

CNS: <u>sedation</u>, decreased mental acuity, depression.
EENT: nasal stuffiness.
CV: MYOCARDITIS, bradycardia, edema, orthostatic hypotension.
GI: DRUG-INDUCED HEPATITIS, diarrhea, dry mouth.
GU: <u>impotence</u>.
Hemat: eosinophilia, hemolytic anemia.
Misc: fever.

INTERACTIONS

Drug-Drug: ■ Additive hypotension with other **antihypertensive agents**, acute ingestion of **alcohol, anesthesia,** and **nitrates** ■ **Amphetamines, barbiturates, tricyclic antidepressants, NSAIDs,** and **phenothiazines** may decrease antihypertensive effect of methyldopa ■ Increased effects and risk of psychoses with **haloperidol** ■ Excess sympathetic stimulation may occur with concurrent use of **MAO inhibitors** or **sympathomimetics** ■ May increase the effects of **tolbutamide** ■ May increase **lithium** toxicity ■ Additive hypotension and CNS toxicity with **levodopa** ■ Additive CNS depression may occur with **alcohol, antihistamines, sedative/hypnotics,** some **antidepressants,** and **opioids** ■ Concurrent use with

nonselective beta-blockers may rarely cause paradoxical hypertension.

ROUTE AND DOSAGE

- **PO (Adults):** 250–500 mg 2–3 times daily (not to exceed 500 mg/day if used with other agents); may be increased q 2 days as needed; usual maintenance dose is 500 mg–2 g/day (not to exceed 3 g/day).
- **PO (Children):** 10 mg/kg/day (300 mg/m²/day); may be increased q 2 days up to 65 mg/kg/day in divided doses (not to exceed 3 g/day).
- **IV (Adults):** 250–500 mg q 6 hr (up to 1 g q 6 hr).
- **IV (Children):** 5–10 mg/kg q 6 hr; up to 65 mg/kg/day in divided doses (not to exceed 3 g/day).

AVAILABILITY

- **Tablets:** 125 mg^Rx, 250 mg^Rx, 500 mg^Rx ■ Cost: *Aldomet*—125 mg $29.85/100, 250 mg $38/100, 500 mg $69.44/100; *generic*—125 mg $9.75–$26.72/100, 250 mg $12.50–$34.01/100, 500 mg $22.50–$62.25/100
- **Oral suspension (orange-pineapple flavor):** 250 mg/5 ml^Rx ■ **Injection:** 250 mg/5 ml in 5- and 10-ml vials^Rx ■ **In combination with:** hydrochlorothiazide (Aldoril)^Rx or chlorothiazide (Aldoclor)^Rx. See Appendix B.

TIME/ACTION PROFILE (antihypertensive effect)

	ONSET	PEAK	DURATION
PO	12–24 hr	4–6 hr	24–48 hr
IV	4–6 hr	unknown	10–16 hr

NURSING IMPLICATIONS

ASSESSMENT

- ❑ Monitor blood pressure and pulse frequently during initial dosage adjustment and periodically throughout therapy. Report significant changes.
- ❑ Monitor frequency of prescription refills to determine compliance.
- ❑ Monitor intake and output ratios and weight and assess for edema daily, especially at beginning of therapy. Report weight gain or edema; sodium and water retention may be treated with diuretics.
- ❑ Assess patient for depression or other alterations in mental status. Notify physician or other health care professional promptly if these symptoms develop.
- ❑ Monitor temperature during therapy. Drug fever may occur shortly after initiation of therapy and may be accompanied by eosinophilia and hepatic function changes. Monitor hepatic function test if unexplained fever occurs.
- ■ *Lab Test Considerations:* Renal and hepatic function and CBC should be monitored before and periodically throughout therapy.
- ❑ Monitor direct Coombs' test before and after 6 and 12 mo of therapy. May cause a positive direct Coombs' test, rarely associated with hemolytic anemia.
- ❑ May cause increased BUN, serum creatinine, potassium, sodium, prolactin, uric acid, AST, ALT, alkaline phosphatase, and bilirubin concentrations.
- ❑ May cause prolonged prothrombin times.
- ❑ May interfere with serum creatinine and AST measurements.

POTENTIAL NURSING DIAGNOSES

- ■ Injury, risk for (Side Effects).
- ■ Knowledge deficit, related to medication regimen (Patient/Family Teaching).
- ■ Noncompliance (Patient/Family Teaching).

IMPLEMENTATION

- ■ **General Info:** Fluid retention and expanded volume may cause tolerance to develop within 2–3 mo after initiation of therapy. Diuretics may be added to regimen at this time to maintain control.
- ❑ Dosage increases should be made with the evening dose to minimize drowsiness.
- ❑ When changing from IV to oral forms, dosage should remain consistent.
- ■ **PO:** Shake suspension before administration.
- ■ **Intermittent Infusion:** Dilute in 100 ml of D5W, 0.9% NaCl, D5/0.9% NaCl, 5% sodium bicarbonate, or Ringer's solution.
- ■ *Rate:* Infuse slowly over 30–60 min.

{ } = Available in Canada only.
†CAPITALS indicate life-threatening; underlines indicate most frequent.

■ **Y-Site Compatibility:** ◆ esmolol ◆ heparin ◆ meperidine ◆ morphine ◆ theophylline.

PATIENT/FAMILY TEACHING

❏ Emphasize the importance of continuing to take this medication, even if feeling well. Instruct patient to take medication at the same time each day; last dose of the day should be taken at bedtime. If a dose is missed, take as soon as remembered but not if almost time for next dose. Do not double doses.

❏ Encourage patient to comply with additional interventions for hypertension (weight reduction, low-sodium diet, smoking cessation, moderation of alcohol consumption, regular exercise, and stress management). Methyldopa controls but does not cure hypertension.

❏ Instruct patient and family on proper technique for monitoring blood pressure. Advise them to check blood pressure at least weekly and to report significant changes.

❏ Inform patient that urine may darken or turn red-black when left standing.

❏ May cause drowsiness. Advise patient to avoid driving or other activities requiring alertness until response to medication is known. Drowsiness usually subsides after 7–10 days of continuous use.

❏ Caution patient to avoid sudden changes in position to decrease orthostatic hypotension.

❏ Advise patient that frequent mouth rinses, good oral hygiene, and sugarless gum or candy may minimize dry mouth. Notify health care professional if dry mouth continues for >2 wk.

❏ Caution patient to avoid concurrent use of alcohol or other CNS depressants.

❏ Advise patient to consult health care professional before taking any cough, cold, or allergy remedies.

❏ Advise patient to notify health care professional of medication regimen before treatment or surgery.

❏ Instruct patient to notify health care professional if fever, muscle aches, or flu-like syndrome occurs.

EVALUATION

Effectiveness of therapy can be demonstrated by: ■ Decrease in blood pressure without appearance of side effects.

NAPROXEN

(na-**prox**-en)
{Apo-Naproxen}, EC-Naprosyn, Naprelan, Napron X, Naprosyn, {Naprosyn-E}, {Naprosyn-SR}, {Naxen}, {Novo-Naprox}, {Novo-Naprox Sodium}, {Nu-Naprox}

NAPROXEN SODIUM

(na-**prox**-en **soe**-dee-um)
Aleve, Anaprox, Anaprox DS, {Apo-Napro-Na}, Apo-Napro-Na DS, Naprelan, {Novo-Naprox Sodium}, {Novo-Naprox Sodium DS}, {Synflex}, {Synflex DS}

CLASSIFICATION(S):
Non-opioid analgesics, Nonsteroidal anti-inflammatory agents

Pregnancy Category B (first trimester)

INDICATIONS

■ Mild to moderate pain ■ Dysmenorrhea ■ Fever ■ Inflammatory disorders, including: ❏ Rheumatoid arthritis ❏ Osteoarthritis.

ACTION

■ Inhibit prostaglandin synthesis. Therapeutic Effects: ■ Decreased pain ■ Reduction of fever ■ Suppression of inflammation.

PHARMACOKINETICS

Absorption: Completely absorbed from the GI tract. Sodium salt (Anaprox) is more rapidly absorbed.

Distribution: Crosses the placenta; enters breast milk in low concentrations.

Protein Binding: >99%

Metabolism and Excretion: Mostly metabolized by the liver.

Half-life: 10–20 hr.

CONTRAINDICATIONS AND PRECAUTIONS

Contraindicated in: ■ Hypersensitivity ■ Cross-sensitivity may occur with other NSAIDs, including aspirin ■ Active GI bleeding ■ Ulcer disease.

Use Cautiously in: ■ Severe cardiovascular, renal, or hepatic disease ■ History of ulcer disease ■ Chronic alcohol use/abuse ■ Pregnancy or lactation (safety not established; avoid using during 2nd half of pregnancy).

ADVERSE REACTIONS AND SIDE EFFECTS†

CNS: <u>dizziness</u>, <u>drowsiness</u>, <u>headache</u>.
EENT: tinnitus.
Resp: dyspnea.
CV: edema, palpitations, tachycardia.
GI: DRUG-INDUCED HEPATITIS, GI BLEEDING, <u>constipation</u>, <u>dyspepsia</u>, <u>nausea</u>, anorexia, diarrhea, discomfort, flatulence, vomiting.
GU: cystitis, hematuria, renal failure.
Derm: photosensitivity, rashes, sweating.
Hemat: blood dyscrasias, prolonged bleeding time.
Misc: allergic reactions including ANAPHYLAXIS.

INTERACTIONS

Drug-Drug: ■ Concurrent use with **aspirin** decreases naproxen blood levels and may decrease effectiveness ■ Increased risk of bleeding with **anticoagulants**, **thrombolytic agents**, **eptifibatide**, **tirofiban**, **cefamandole**, **cefotetan**, **cefoperazone**, **valproic acid**, **clopidogrel**, **ticlopidine**, **plicamycin** ■ Additive adverse GI side effects with **aspirin**, **corticosteroids**, and other **NSAIDs** ■ **Probenecid** increases levels and may increase toxicity ■ Increased risk of photosensitivity with other **photosensitizing agents** ■ May increase the risk of toxicity from **methotrexate**, **antineoplastic agents**, or **radiation therapy** ■ May increase serum levels and risk of toxicity from **lithium** ■ Increased risk of adverse renal effects with **cyclosporine** or chronic use of **acetaminophen** ■ May decrease response to **antihypertensives** or **diuretics** ■ May increase risk of hypoglycemia with **insulin** or **oral hypoglycemic agents**.

ROUTE AND DOSAGE

275 mg naproxen sodium is equivalent to 250 mg naproxen.

□ **Anti-inflammatory/Analgesic/Antidysmenorrheal**
■ **PO (Adults):** *Naproxen*—250–500 mg naproxen bid (up to 1.5 g/day). *Delayed-release naproxen*—375–500 mg twice daily. *Naproxen sodium*—275–550 mg twice daily (up to 1.65 g/day).
■ **PO (Children):** 5 mg/kg/day twice daily as naproxen suspension.

□ **Antigout**
■ **PO (Adults):** *Naproxen*—750 mg naproxen initially, then 250 mg q 8 hr. *Naproxen sodium*—825 mg initially, then 275 mg q 8 hr.

□ **OTC Use**
■ **PO (Adults):** 200 mg q 8–12 hr or 400 mg followed by 200 mg q 12 hr (not to exceed 600 mg/24 hr).
■ **PO (Geriatric Patients >65 yr):** Not to exceed 200 mg q 12 hr.

AVAILABILITY

□ **Naproxen (generic available)**
■ *Tablets (Naprosyn, {Apo-Naproxen, Naxen, Novo-Naprox, Nu-Naprox}):* {125 mg^{Rx}}, 250 mg^{Rx}, 375 mg^{Rx}, 500 mg^{Rx} ■ *Controlled-release tablets (Naprelan):* 375 mg^{Rx}, 500 mg^{Rx} ■ *Delayed-release tablets (EC-Naprosyn, {Naprosyn-E}):* {250 mg^{Rx}}, 375 mg^{Rx}, 500 mg^{Rx} ■ *Extended-release tablets {Naprosyn-SR}:* {750 mg^{Rx}} ■ *Oral suspension (Naprosyn):* 125 mg/5 ml^{Rx} ■ *Suppositories (Naprosyn, {Naxen}):* {500 mg^{Rx}}.

□ **Naproxen Sodium**
■ *Tablets (Aleve, Anaprox, Anaprox DS, {Apo-Napro-Na, Novo-Naprox Sodium, Novo-Naprox Sodium DS, Synaflex, Synaflex DS}):* 220 mg^{OTC}, 275 mg^{Rx}, 550 mg^{Rx}.

TIME/ACTION PROFILE

	ONSET	PEAK	DURATION
PO (analgesic)	1 hr	Unknown	up to 7 hr
PO (anti-inflammatory)	14 days	2–4 wk	Unknown

{ } = Available in Canada only.
†CAPITALS indicate life-threatening; <u>underlines</u> indicate most frequent.

NURSING IMPLICATIONS

ASSESSMENT

- **General Info:** Patients who have asthma, aspirin-induced allergy, and nasal polyps are at increased risk for developing hypersensitivity reactions. Assess for rhinitis, asthma, and urticaria.
- **Pain:** Assess pain (note type, location, and intensity) prior to and 1–2 hr following administration.
- **Arthritis:** Assess pain and range of motion prior to and 1–2 hr following administration.
- **Fever:** Monitor temperature; note signs associated with fever (diaphoresis, tachycardia, malaise).
- *Lab Test Considerations:* BUN, serum creatinine, CBC, and liver function tests should be evaluated periodically in patients receiving prolonged courses of therapy.
- Serum potassium, BUN, serum creatinine, alkaline phosphatase, LDH, AST, and ALT tests may show increased levels. Blood glucose, hemoglobin, and hematocrit concentrations, leukocyte and platelet counts, and CCr may be decreased.
- Bleeding time may be prolonged up to 4 days following discontinuation of therapy.
- May alter test results for urine 5-HIAA and urine steroid determinations.

POTENTIAL NURSING DIAGNOSES

- Pain (Indications).
- Impaired physical mobility (Indications).
- Knowledge deficit, related to medication regimen (Patient/Family Teaching).

IMPLEMENTATION

- **General Info:** Administration in higher than recommended doses does not provide increased effectiveness but may cause increased side effects.
- Coadministration with opioid analgesics may have additive analgesic effects and may permit lower opioid doses.
- Analgesic is more effective if given before pain becomes severe.
- **PO:** For rapid initial effect, administer 30 min before or 2 hr after meals. May be administered with food, milk, or antacids to decrease GI irritation. Food slows but does not reduce the extent of absorption. Do not mix suspension with antacid or other liquid prior to administration.
- **Dysmenorrhea:** Administer as soon as possible after the onset of menses. Prophylactic treatment has not been shown to be effective.

PATIENT/FAMILY TEACHING

- Advise patient to take this medication with a full glass of water and to remain in an upright position for 15–30 min after administration.
- Instruct patient to take medication exactly as directed. If a dose is missed, it should be taken as soon as remembered but not if almost time for the next dose. Do not double doses.
- May cause drowsiness or dizziness. Advise patient to avoid driving or other activities requiring alertness until response to the medication is known.
- Caution patient to avoid the concurrent use of alcohol, aspirin, acetaminophen, or other OTC medications without consulting health care professional. Use of naproxen with 3 or more glasses of alcohol per day may increase risk of GI bleeding.
- Advise patient to inform health care professional of medication regimen prior to treatment or surgery.
- Caution patient to wear sunscreen and protective clothing to prevent photosensitivity reactions.
- Instruct patients not to take OTC naproxen preparations for more than 3 days for fever and to consult health care professional if symptoms persist or worsen.
- Advise patient to consult health care professional if rash, itching, visual disturbances, tinnitus, weight gain, edema, black stools, persistent headache, or influenza-like syndrome (chills, fever, muscle aches, pain) occurs.

EVALUATION

Effectiveness of therapy can be demonstrated by:■ Relief of pain ■ Improved joint mobility. Partial arthritic relief is usually seen within 2 wk, but maximum effectiveness may require 2–4 wk of continuous therapy. Patients who do not respond to one NSAID may respond to another ■ Reduction of fever.

OXYCODONE

(ox-i-**koe**-done)

Endocodone, Oxycontin, OxyFAST, OxyIR, Percolone, Roxicodone, Roxicodone SR, {Supeudol}

OXYCODONE/ACETAMINOPHEN

(See also acetaminophen monograph on page 3.)

{Endocet}, {Oxycocet}, Percocet, {Percocet}, Roxicet, Roxilox, Tylox

OXYCODONE/ASPIRIN

(See also salicylates monograph on page 903.)

{Endodan}, {Oxycodan}, Percodan, Percodan-Demi, Roxiprin

CLASSIFICATION(S):
Opioid analgesic (agonist)

Pregnancy Category C (oxycodone alone)

INDICATIONS

■ Management of moderate to severe pain.

ACTION

■ Bind to opiate receptors in the CNS ■ Alter the perception of and response to painful stimuli, while producing generalized CNS depression. Therapeutic Effects: ■ Decreased pain.

PHARMACOKINETICS

Absorption: Well absorbed from the GI tract.
Distribution: Widely distributed. Cross the placenta; enter breast milk.
Metabolism and Excretion: Mostly metabolized by the liver.
Half-life: 2–3 hr.

CONTRAINDICATIONS AND PRECAUTIONS

Contraindicated in: ■ Hypersensitivity ■ Pregnancy or lactation (avoid chronic use) ■ Some products contain alcohol or bisulfites and should be avoided in patients with known intolerance or hypersensitivity.

Use Cautiously in: ■ Head trauma ■ Increased intracranial pressure ■ Severe renal, hepatic, or pulmonary disease ■ Hypothyroidism ■ Adrenal insufficiency ■ Alcoholism ■ Geriatric or debilitated patients (initial dosage reduction recommended) ■ Undiagnosed abdominal pain ■ Prostatic hypertrophy.

ADVERSE REACTIONS AND SIDE EFFECTS

CNS: <u>confusion</u>, <u>sedation</u>, dizziness, dysphoria, euphoria, floating feeling, hallucinations, headache, unusual dreams.
EENT: blurred vision, diplopia, miosis.
Resp: RESPIRATORY DEPRESSION .
CV: orthostatic hypotension.
GI: <u>constipation</u>, dry mouth, nausea, vomiting.
GU: urinary retention.
Derm: flushing, sweating.
Misc: physical dependence, psychological dependence, tolerance.

INTERACTIONS

Drug-Drug: ■ Use with caution in patients receiving **MAO inhibitors** (may result in unpredictable reactions—decrease initial dose of oxycodone to 25% of usual dose) ■ Additive CNS depression with **alcohol**, **antihistamines**, and **sedative/hypnotics** ■ Administration of **partial-antagonist opioid analgesics** may precipitate withdrawal in physically dependent patients ■ **Nalbuphine, buprenorphine, dezocine,** or **pentazocine** may decrease analgesia.

ROUTE AND DOSAGE

Larger doses may be required during chronic therapy. Consider cumulative effects of additional acetaminophen/aspirin; if toxic levels are exceeded, change to pure oxycodone product.

■ **PO (Adults ≥50 kg):** 5–10 mg q 3–4 hr initially, as needed. Controlled-release tablets (Oxycontin) may be given q 12 hr.
■ **PO (Adults <50 kg or Children):** 0.2 mg/kg q 3–4 hr initially, as needed.
■ **Rect (Adults):** 10–40 mg 3–4 times daily initially, as needed.

{ } = Available in Canada only.
†CAPITALS indicate life-threatening; <u>underlines</u> indicate most frequent.

AVAILABILITY

☐ Oxycodone

■ *Tablets:* 5 mg (Percolone, Roxicodone, Supeudol)^{Rx} ■ Cost: *Percolone—*$68.75/100; *Roxicodone—*$31.04/100; *generic—*$27.00–41.99/100 ■ *Immediate-release capsules:* 5 mg (OxyIR)^{Rx} ■ *Controlled-release tablets:* 10 mg^{Rx}, 20^{Rx}, 40 mg^{Rx}, 80 mg (Oxycontin, Roxicodone SR)^{Rx}, 160 mg (Oxycontin) ■ Cost: *Oxycontin—*10 mg $117.10/100, 20 mg $224.11/100, 40 mg $397.66/100, 80 mg $747.79/100; *Roxicodone SR—* ■ *Oral solution (burgundy cherry):* 5 mg/5 ml in 500-ml bottle (Roxicodone)^{Rx} ■ Cost: 41.65/500 ml

■ *Concentrated oral solution:* 20 mg/ml in 30-ml bottle with dropper (Roxicodone Intensol, OxyFAST)^{Rx} ■ Cost: *Roxicodone Intensol—*$40.56/30 ml; *OxyFAST—*$33.75/30 ml

☐ Oxycodone/Acetaminophen

■ *Tablets:* 2.5 mg oxycodone with 325 mg acetaminophen (Percocet 2.5)^{Rx}, 5 mg oxycodone with 325 mg acetaminophen (Endocet, Oxycet, Percocet, Roxicet)^{Rx}, 7.5 mg oxycodone with 500 mg acetaminophen (Percocet 7.5)^{Rx}, 10 mg oxycodone with 650 mg acetaminophen (Percocet 10)^{Rx} ■ Cost: *Endocet—*$25.73/100,*Percocet 5—*$83.75/100, *Roxicet—*$25.73/100,

■ *Capsules:* 5 mg oxycodone with 500 mg acetaminophen (Roxilox, Tylox)^{Rx} ■ Cost: *Roxilox—*$57.72/100; *Tylox—*$87.35/100

■ *Caplets:* 5 mg oxycodone with 500 mg acetaminophen (Roxicet 5/500)^{Rx} ■ Cost: $57.60/100 ■ *Oral solution (mint):* 5 mg oxycodone with 325 mg acetaminophen/5 ml (Roxicet Solution) in 500-ml bottles^{Rx} ■ Cost: $37.37/500 ml.

☐ Oxycodone/Aspirin

■ *Tablets:* 2.44 mg oxycodone with 325 mg aspirin (Percodan-Demi)^{Rx}, 4.88 mg oxycodone with 325 mg aspirin (Endodan, Oxycodan, Percodan, Roxiprin)^{Rx}.

TIME/ACTION PROFILE (analgesic effects)

	ONSET	PEAK	DURATION
PO	10–15 min	60–90 min	3–6 hr
PO-CR	10–15 min	3 hr	12 hr

NURSING IMPLICATIONS

ASSESSMENT

☐ Assess type, location, and intensity of pain prior to and 1 hr (peak) after administration. When titrating opioid doses, increases of 25–50% should be administered until there is either a 50% reduction in the patient's pain rating on a numerical or visual analogue scale or the patient reports satisfactory pain relief. A repeat dose can be safely administered at the time of the peak if previous dose is ineffective and side effects are minimal.

☐ Patients taking controlled-release tablets should also be given supplemental short-acting opioid doses for breakthrough pain.

☐ An equianalgesic chart (see Appendix C) should be used when changing routes or when changing from one opioid to another.

☐ Assess blood pressure, pulse, and respirations before and periodically during administration. If respiratory rate is <10/min, assess level of sedation. Physical stimulation may be sufficient to prevent significant hypoventilation. Dose may need to be decreased by 25–50%. Initial drowsiness will diminish with continued use.

☐ Prolonged use may lead to physical and psychological dependence and tolerance. This should not prevent patient from receiving adequate analgesia. Most patients who receive oxycodone for pain do not develop psychological dependence. Progressively higher doses may be required to relieve pain with long-term therapy.

☐ Assess bowel function routinely. Prevention of constipation should be instituted with increased intake of fluids and bulk, and laxatives to minimize constipating effects. Stimulant laxatives should be administered routinely if opioid use exceeds 2–3 days, unless contraindicated.

■ *Lab Test Considerations:* May increase plasma amylase and lipase levels.

■ *Toxicity and Overdose:* If an opioid antagonist is required to reverse respiratory depression or coma, naloxone (Narcan) is the antidote. Dilute the 0.4-mg ampule of naloxone in 10 ml of 0.9% NaCl and administer 0.5 ml (0.02 mg) by direct IV push every 2 min. For children and patients weighing <40 kg, dilute 0.1 mg of naloxone in 10 ml of 0.9%

NaCl for a concentration of 10 mcg/ml and administer 0.5 mcg/kg every 2 min. Titrate dose to avoid withdrawal, seizures, and severe pain.

POTENTIAL NURSING DIAGNOSES

■ Pain (Indications).

■ Sensory-perceptual alterationsvisual, auditory (Side Effects).

■ Injury, risk for (Side Effects).

IMPLEMENTATION

■ **General Info:** Explain therapeutic value of medication prior to administration to enhance the analgesic effect.

❑ Regularly administered doses may be more effective than prn administration. Analgesic is more effective if given before pain becomes severe.

❑ Coadministration with nonopioid analgesics may have additive analgesic effects and may permit lower doses.

❑ Medication should be discontinued gradually after long-term use to prevent withdrawal symptoms.

■ **PO:** May be administered with food or milk to minimize GI irritation.

❑ Administer solution with properly calibrated measuring device.

❑ Controlled-release tablets should be swallowed whole; do not crush, break, or chew.

■ **Controlled Release:** Dose should be based on 24-hr opioid requirement determined with short-acting opioids then converted to controlled-release form.

PATIENT/FAMILY TEACHING

❑ Instruct patient on how and when to ask for pain medication.

❑ Medication may cause drowsiness or dizziness. Advise patient to call for assistance when ambulating or smoking. Caution patient to avoid driving and other activities requiring alertness until response to medication is known.

❑ Advise patients taking Oxycontin tablets that empty matrix tablets may appear in stool.

❑ Advise patient to make position changes slowly to minimize orthostatic hypotension.

❑ Advise patient to avoid concurrent use of alcohol or other CNS depressants with this medication.

❑ Encourage patient to turn, cough, and breathe deeply every 2 hr to prevent atelectasis.

EVALUATION

Effectiveness of therapy can be demonstrated by: ■ Decrease in severity of pain without a significant alteration in level of consciousness or respiratory status.

QUININE
(**kwi**-nine)

CLASSIFICATION(S):
Anti-infective agents (antimalarial)

Pregnancy Category X

INDICATIONS

■ Combination with other agents in the treatment of chloroquine-resistant malaria. **Unlabeled Uses:** ■ Prophylaxis and treatment of nocturnal recumbency leg cramps, including those associated with arthritis, diabetes, varicose veins, thrombophlebitis, arteriosclerosis, and static foot deformities.

ACTION

■ Disrupts metabolism of the erythrocytic phase of *Plasmodium falciparum* ■ Increases the refractory period of skeletal muscle, increases the distribution of calcium within muscle fibers, decreases the excitability of motor end-plate regions, resulting in decreased response to repetitive nerve stimulation and acetylcholine. Therapeutic Effects: ■ Death of *P. falciparum* ■ Decreased severity of leg cramps.

PHARMACOKINETICS

Absorption: Rapidly and almost completely (80%) absorbed following oral administration.

Distribution: Varies with condition and patient; does not enter CSF well. Crosses the placenta and enters breast milk.

Protein Binding: >90% in patients with cerebral malaria, pregnant women and children, 85–

90% in patients with uncomplicated malaria, 70% in healthy adults.

Metabolism and Excretion: >80% metabolized by the liver; metabolites have less activity than quinine; metabolites excreted in urine. 20% excreted unchanged in urine. Excretion increased in acidic urine.

Half-life: 11 hr (increased in patients with malaria).

CONTRAINDICATIONS AND PRECAUTIONS

Contraindicated in: ■ Hypersensitivity ■ Pregnancy or lactation.

Use Cautiously in: ■ Recurrent or interrupted malaria therapy ■ History of arrhythmias, especially QT prolongation ■ G6PD deficiency ■ Hypoglycemia ■ Myasthenia gravis ■ History of thrombocytopenic purpura.

ADVERSE REACTIONS AND SIDE EFFECTS†

GI: <u>abdominal cramps/pain</u>, <u>diarrhea</u>, <u>nausea</u>, <u>vomiting</u>, hepatotoxicity.
Derm: rash.
Endo: hypoglycemia.
Hemat: bleeding, blood dyscrasias.
Misc: <u>cinchonism</u>, hypersensitivity reactions including fever and HEMOLYTIC UREMIC SYNDROME.

INTERACTIONS

Drug-Drug: ■ May increase serum **digoxin** levels ■ May increase the risk of hemolytic, ototoxic, or neurotoxic reactions when used concurrently with **agents sharing these toxicities** ■ Concurrent use with **quinidine** may increase the risk of adverse cardiovascular reactions ■ May increase the risk of bleeding with **warfarin** ■ Concurrent use with **mefloquine** increases the risk of seizures and adverse cardiovascular reactions.

ROUTE AND DOSAGE

■ **PO (Adults):** *Malaria*—600–650 mg q 8 hr for 3 days (7 days in southeast Asia) with tetracycline or doxycycline or sulfadoxine/pyrimethamine or clindamycin; *leg cramps (unlabeled)*—200–300 mg at bedtime, if needed an additional 200–300 mg may be given with supper.

■ **PO (Children):** 8.3 mg/kg q 8 hr for 3 days (7 days in southeast Asia) with tetracycline or

doxycycline (if child is over 8 yr) or sulfadoxine/pyramethamine or clindamycin.

AVAILABILITY

■ *Capsules:* 200 mg^Rx, 300 mg^Rx, 325 mg^Rx ■ Cost: 325 mg $5.15–$8.28/30
■ *Tablets:* 260 mg^Rx, 325 mg^Rx ■ Cost: 260 mg $3.89–$3.95/30.

TIME/ACTION PROFILE (antimalarial blood levels)

	ONSET	PEAK	DURATION
PO	unknown	3.2–5.9 hr	8 hr

NURSING IMPLICATIONS

ASSESSMENT

■ **Malaria:** Assess patient for improvement in signs and symptoms of condition daily throughout therapy.
■ **Nocturnal recumbency leg cramps:** Assess frequency and severity of nocturnal leg cramps. If cramps do not occur for several consecutive nights, may be discontinued to determine if continued use is required.
■ *Lab Test Considerations:* May cause elevated levels of urinary 17-ketogenic steroids when metyrapone or Zimmerman method is used.
■ *Toxicity and Overdose:* Plasma quinine levels of >10 mcg/ml may cause tinnitus and impaired hearing.
❑ Signs of toxicity or cinchonism include tinnitus, headache, nausea, and slightly disturbed vision; usually disappear rapidly upon discontinuing quinine.

POTENTIAL NURSING DIAGNOSES

■ Infection, risk for (Indications).
■ Pain, chronic (Indications).
■ Knowledge deficit, related to medication regimen (Patient/Family Teaching).

IMPLEMENTATION

■ **PO:** Administer with or after meals to minimize GI distress. Aluminum-containing antacids will decrease and delay absorption; avoid concurrent use.

PATIENT/FAMILY TEACHING

❑ Instruct patient to take medication exactly as directed and continue full course of therapy, even if feeling better. Missed doses should be taken as soon as remembered, unless almost time for the next dose. Do not double doses or take more than recommended.

❑ Review methods of minimizing exposure to mosquitoes with patients receiving chloroquine prophylactically (use repellent, wear long-sleeved shirt and long trousers, use screen or netting).

❑ Quinine may cause visual changes. Caution patient to avoid driving or other activities requiring alertness until response to medication is known.

❑ May cause diarrhea, nausea, stomach cramps or pain, vomiting, or ringing in the ears. Advise patient to notify health care professional promptly if these become pronounced.

❑ Advise patient to stop quinine and notify health care professional of any evidence of allergy (flushing, itching, rash, fever, stomach pain, difficult breathing, ringing in the ears, visual problems).

EVALUATION

Effectiveness of therapy can be demonstrated by: ■ Prevention of or improvement in signs and symptoms of malaria ■ Decrease in frequency and severity of nocturnal redundancy leg cramps.

ROSIGLITAZONE
(roe-zi-**glit**-a-zone)
Avandia

CLASSIFICATION(S):
Antidiabetic agents (thiazolidinedione)

Pregnancy Category C

INDICATIONS

■ Used as an adjunct to diet and exercise in the management of type 2 diabetes mellitus; may also be used with metformin when the combination of diet, exercise, and metformin does not achieve glycemic control.

ACTION

■ Improves sensitivity to insulin by acting as an agonist at receptor sites involved in insulin re-

sponsiveness and subsequent glucose production and utilization ■ Requires insulin for activity. Therapeutic Effects: ■ Decreased insulin resistance, resulting in glycemic control without hypoglycemia.

PHARMACOKINETICS

Absorption: Well absorbed (99%) following oral administration.
Distribution: Unknown.
Protein Binding: 99.8% bound to plasma proteins.
Metabolism and Excretion: Entirely metabolized by the liver.
Half-life: 3.2–3.6 hr (increased in liver disease).

CONTRAINDICATIONS AND PRECAUTIONS

Contraindicated in: ■ Hypersensitivity ■ Pregnancy or lactation (not recommended for use during pregnancy or lactation; insulin should be used) ■ Children <18 yr or with type 1 diabetes (requires insulin for activity) ■ Diabetic ketoacidosis ■ Clinical evidence of active liver disease or increased ALT (>2.5 times upper limit of normal).
Use Cautiously in: ■ Edema ■ Congestive heart failure (avoid use in moderate to severe CHF unless benefits outweigh risks) ■ Hepatic impairment ■ Women with child-bearing potential (may restore ovulation and risk of pregnancy).

ADVERSE REACTIONS AND SIDE EFFECTS†

CV: edema.
Hemat: anemia.
Metab: increased total cholesterol, LDL and HDL, weight gain.

INTERACTIONS

Drug-Drug: ■ None known.

ROUTE AND DOSAGE

■ **PO (Adults):** 4 mg as a single dose once daily or 2 mg twice daily; after 12 weeks, may be increased if necessary to 8 mg once daily or 4 mg twice daily.

AVAILABILITY

■ *Tablets:* 2 mg^{Rx}, 4 mg^{Rx}, 8 mg^{Rx}.

TIME/ACTION PROFILE (effects on blood glucose)

	ONSET	PEAK	DURATION
PO	unknown	unknown	12–24 hr

NURSING IMPLICATIONS

ASSESSMENT

❑ Observe patient taking current insulin for signs and symptoms of hypoglycemic reactions (sweating, hunger, weakness, dizziness, tremor, tachycardia, anxiety).

■ *Lab Test Considerations:* Serum glucose and glycosylated hemoglobin should be monitored periodically throughout therapy to evaluate effectiveness of treatment.

❑ Monitor CBC with differential periodically throughout therapy. May cause decrease in hemoglobin, hematocrit, and WBC, usually during the first 4–8 wk of therapy; then levels stabilize.

❑ Monitor AST and ALT every 2 months during the first 12 months of therapy and periodically thereafter or if jaundice or symptoms of hepatic dysfunction occur. May cause irreversible elevations in AST and ALT or hepatic failure (rare). If ALT increases to >3 times the upper limit of normal, recheck ALT promptly. Discontinue rosiglitazone if ALT remains >3 times normal.

❑ May cause increases in total cholesterol, LDL, and HDL and decreases in free fatty acids.

POTENTIAL NURSING DIAGNOSES

■ Nutrition: altered, more than body requirements (Indications).

■ Knowledge deficit (Patient/Family Teaching).

IMPLEMENTATION

■ **General Info:** Patients stabilized on a diabetic regimen who are exposed to stress, fever, trauma, infection, or surgery may require administration of insulin.

■ **PO:** May be administered with or without meals.

PATIENT/FAMILY TEACHING

❑ Instruct patient to take medication exactly as directed. If dose for 1 day is missed, do not double dose the next day.

❑ Explain to patient that this medication controls hyperglycemia but does not cure diabetes. Therapy is long-term.

❑ Review signs of hypoglycemia and hyperglycemia with patient. If hypoglycemia occurs, advise patient to take a glass of orange juice or 2–3 tsp of sugar, honey, or corn syrup dissolved in water and notify health care professional.

❑ Encourage patient to follow prescribed diet, medication, and exercise regimen to prevent hypoglycemic or hyperglycemic episodes.

❑ Instruct patient in proper testing of serum glucose and ketones. These tests should be closely monitored during periods of stress or illness and health care professional notified if significant changes occur.

❑ Advise patient to notify health care professional immediately if signs of hepatic dysfunction (nausea, vomiting, abdominal pain, fatigue, anorexia, dark urine, jaundice) occur.

❑ Insulin is the preferred method of controlling blood sugar during pregnancy. Counsel female patients that higher doses of oral contraceptives or a form of contraception other than oral contraceptives may be required and to notify health care professional promptly if pregnancy is planned or suspected.

❑ Advise patient to inform health care professional of medication regimen prior to treatment or surgery.

❑ Advise patient to carry a form of sugar (sugar packets, candy) and identification describing disease process and medication regimen at all times.

❑ Emphasize the importance of routine follow-up exams.

EVALUATION

Effectiveness of therapy can be demonstrated by:■ Control of blood glucose levels.

SECTION III
Drug Update 2001

BALSALAZIDE
(ba-**sal**-a-zide)
Colazal

CLASSIFICATION(S):
Nonsteroidal anti-inflammatory agents
(gastrointestinal/local)

Pregnancy Category B

INDICATIONS

■ Treatment of mild to moderately active ulcerative colitis.

ACTION

■ Drug is metabolized in the colon to mesalamine (5-aminosalicylic acid), which is a local anti-inflammatory. Therapeutic Effects: ■ Reduction in the symptoms of ulcerative colitis.

PHARMACOKINETICS

Absorption: Absorption is low and variable; drug is delivered intact to the colon.
Distribution: Mostly delivered intact to the colon; remainder of distribution unknown.
Protein Binding: ≥99%
Metabolism and Excretion: Following delivery to the colon, bacteria break balsalazide down into mesalamine (5-aminosalicylic acid) and an inactive metabolite; mostly excreted in feces.
Half-life: *Mesalamine*—12 hr (range 2–15 hr).

CONTRAINDICATIONS AND PRECAUTIONS

Contraindicated in: ■ Hypersensitivity to salicylates or other metabolites.
Use Cautiously in: ■ Pyloric stenosis (may have prolonged gastric retention of capsules) ■ Pregnancy (use only if clearly needed) ■ Lactation and children (safety not established).

ADVERSE REACTIONS AND SIDE EFFECTS

GI: abdominal pain, diarrhea.

INTERACTIONS

Drug-Drug: ■ None known.

ROUTE AND DOSAGE

■ **PO (Adults):** 2.25 g three times daily (three 750 mg capsules three times daily) for 8–12 wks.

AVAILABILITY

■ *Capsules:* 750 mg

TIME/ACTION PROFILE (decreased symptoms)

	ONSET	PEAK	DURATION
PO	UK	up to 8 wk	UK

NURSING IMPLICATIONS

ASSESSMENT

❑ Assess abdominal pain and frequency, quantity, and consistency of stools at the beginning of and throughout therapy.
❑ Assess patient for allergy to salicylates.
■ *Lab Test Considerations:* May cause elevated AST, ALT, serum alkaline phosphatase, gamma glutamyl transpepsidase (GGT), LDH, and bilirubin.

POTENTIAL NURSING DIAGNOSES

■ Pain (Indications).
■ Diarrhea (Indications).
■ Knowledge deficit, related to medication regimen (Patient/Family Teaching).

{ } = Available in Canada only.
†CAPITALS indicate life-threatening; underlines indicate most frequent.

IMPLEMENTATION

- **PO:** Administer 3 capsules three times a day for 8–12 wks.

PATIENT/FAMILY TEACHING

- ❑ Instruct patient on the correct method of administration. Advise patient to take medication as directed, even if feeling better. If a dose is missed, it should be taken as soon as remembered unless almost time for next dose.
- ❑ Advise patient to notify health care professional if skin rash, difficulty breathing, or hives occur.
- ❑ Instruct patient to notify health care professional if symptoms do not improve after 1–2 mo of therapy.

EVALUATION

Clinical response to therapy can be evaluated by: ■ Decrease in diarrhea and abdominal pain in patients with ulcerative colitis.

COLESEVELAM
(koe-le-**sev**-e-lam)
Welchol

CLASSIFICATION(S):
Lipid-lowering agents (bile acid sequestrant)

Pregnancy Category B

INDICATIONS

■ Adjunctive therapy to diet and exercise for the reduction of LDL cholesterol in patients with primary hypercholesterolemia; may be used alone or in combination with and hepatic hydroxymethylglutaryl coenzyme A (HMG-CoA) reductase inhibitor.

ACTION

■ Binds bile acids in the GI tract ■ Result in increased clearance of cholesterol. Therapeutic Effects: ■ Decreased cholesterol.

PHARMACOKINETICS

Absorption: Not absorbed; action is primarily local in the GI tract.
Distribution: UK.
Metabolism and Excretion: UK.
Half-life: UK.

CONTRAINDICATIONS AND PRECAUTIONS

Contraindicated in: ■ Hypersensitivity ■ Bowel obstruction.
Use Cautiously in: ■ Triglycerides >300 mg/dL ■ Dysphagia, swallowing disorders, severe GI molitlity disorders, or major GI tract surgery. ■ Pregnancy, lactation, or children (safety not established).

ADVERSE REACTIONS AND SIDE EFFECTS

GI: constipation, dyspepsia.

INTERACTIONS

Drug-Drug: ■ May decrease blood levels of sustained-release form of **verapamil**.

ROUTE AND DOSAGE

■ **PO (Adults):** 3 tablets twice daily or 6 tablets once daily; may be increased to 7 tablets daily.

AVAILABILITY

■ **Tablets:** 625 mg.

TIME/ACTION PROFILE (cholesterol-lowering effect)

	ONSET	PEAK	DURATION
PO	24–48 hr	2 wk	UK

NURSING IMPLICATIONS

ASSESSMENT

- ❑ Obtain a diet history, especially in regard to fat consumption.
- ■ *Lab Test Considerations:* Serum total cholesterol, LDL, and triglyceride levels should be evaluated before initiating, and periodically throughout, the therapy.

POTENTIAL NURSING DIAGNOSES

- ■ Constipation (Side Effects).
- ■ Knowledge deficit, related to diet and medication regimen (Patient/Family Teaching).
- ■ Noncompliance (Patient/Family Teaching).

IMPLEMENTATION

- ■ **PO:** Administer once or twice daily with meals. Colesevelam should be taken with a liquid.

PATIENT/FAMILY TEACHING

❏ Instruct patient to take medication exactly as directed; do not skip doses or double up on missed doses.

❏ Advise patient that this medication should be used in conjunction with diet restrictions (fat, cholesterol, carbohydrates, alcohol), exercise, and cessation of smoking.

EVALUATION

Effectiveness of therapy can be demonstrated by: ■ Decrease in serum total cholesterol, low-density lipoprotein (LDL) cholesterol, and apolipoprotein levels.

DOCOSANOL
(doe-**koe**-sa-nole)
Abreva

CLASSIFICATION(S):
Antiviral agents (topical)

Pregnancy Category B

INDICATIONS

■ Treatment of recurrent oral-facial herpes simplex (cold sores, fever blisters).

ACTION

■ Prevents herpes simplex virus from entering cells by preventing viral particles from fusing with cell membranes. Therapeutic Effects: ■ Reduced healing time ■ Decreased duration of symptoms (pain, burning, itching, tingling).

PHARMACOKINETICS

Absorption: UK.
Distribution: UK.
Metabolism and Excretion: UK.
Half-life: UK.

CONTRAINDICATIONS AND PRECAUTIONS

Contraindicated in: ■ Hypersensitivity to docosanol or any other components of the formulation (benzyl alcohol, mineral oil, propylene glycol, or sucrose).

Use Cautiously in: ■ Children <12 yr (safety not established) ■ Pregnancy (use only if clearly needed).

ADVERSE REACTIONS AND SIDE EFFECTS

All local reactions occurred at site of application.
Local: acne, skin, itching, rash.

INTERACTIONS

Drug-Drug: ■ None significant.

ROUTE AND DOSAGE

■ **Topical (Adults and Children ≥12 yr):** Apply small amount 5 times daily to sores on lips or face until healed.

AVAILABILITY

■ *Cream:* 10% cream in 2 g tubes^OTC ■ Cost: $16.99/2 g tube.

TIME/ACTION PROFILE

	ONSET	PEAK	DURATION
Topical	UK	UK	UK

NURSING IMPLICATIONS

ASSESSMENT

❏ Assess skin lesions prior to and periodically throughout therapy.

POTENTIAL NURSING DIAGNOSES

■ Skin integrity, impaired (Indications).
■ Infection transmission, high risk for (Indications).
■ Knowledge deficit, related to disease processes and medication regimen (Patient/Family Teaching).

IMPLEMENTATION

■ **Topical:** Cream should be applied to lesions 5 times daily starting at the first sign of a sore or blister.

PATIENT/FAMILY TEACHING

❏ Instruct patient on correct technique for application of docosanol. Cream should only be applied to lips and face. Avoid application in or near eyes. Emphasize handwashing following application, or touching lesions to prevent spread to others or to other areas of the body.

❏ Advise patient to begin application of docosanol at the first sign of a sore or blister, even during prodromal stage (feeling of burning, itching, tingling or numbness).

❏ Inform patient that docosanol reduces duration of herpes simplex virus episodes but does not cure virus. Viral reactivation may be triggered by ultraviolet radiation or sun exposure, stress, fatigue, chilling, and windburn. Other possible triggers include fever, injury, menstruation, dental work, and infectious diseases (cold, flu).

❏ Advise patient to notify health care professional if lesions do not heal in 14 days or if fever, rash, or swollen lymph nodes occur.

EVALUATION

Clinical response to therapy can be evaluated by: ■ Reduction in duration of symptoms (pain, burning, itching, tingling) of herpes simplex virus episodes.

DOFETILIDE
(doe-**fet**-il-ide)
Tikosyn

CLASSIFICATION(S):
Antiarrhythmic agents (Group III)

Pregnancy Category C

INDICATIONS

■ Maintenance of normal sinus rhythm (delay in time to recurrence of atrial fibrillation/atrial flutter [AF/AFl]) in patients with AF/AFl of greater than 1 week duration, and who have been converted to normal sinus rhythm. ■ For the conversion of atrial fibrillation and atrial flutter to normal sinus rhythm.

ACTION

■ Blocks cardiac ion channels responsible for transport of potassium ■ Increases monophasic action potential duration ■ Increases effective refractory period. Therapeutic Effects: ■ Prevention of recurrent AF/AFl ■ Conversion of AF/AFl to normal sinus rhythm.

PHARMACOKINETICS

Absorption: Well absorbed (>90%) following oral administration.
Distribution: Unknown.
Metabolism and Excretion: 80% excreted by kidneys via cationic renal secretion, mostly as unchanged drug; 20% excreted as inactive metabolites; some metabolism in the liver via cytochrome P450 system (CYP 3A4 isoenzyme).
Half-life: 10 hr

CONTRAINDICATIONS AND PRECAUTIONS

Contraindicated in: ■ Hypersensitivity ■ Congenital or acquired prolonged QT syndromes ■ Baseline QT interval or QTc of >440 msec (500 msec in patients with ventricular conduction abnormalities) ■ Creatinine clearance (CCr) <20 ml/min ■ Concurrent use of verapamil or agents that inhibit the renal cation transport system including cimetidine, ketoconazole, trimethoprim, megestrol or prochlorperazine ■ Lactation (use should be avoided).
Use Cautiously in: ■ Underlying electrolyte abnormalities (increased risk of serious arrhythmias; correct prior to administration) ■ CCr 20–60 ml/min (dosage reduction recommended) ■ Severe hepatic impairment ■ Pregnancy (use only when benefit to patient outweighs potential risk to fetus) ■ Children <18 yr (safety not established).

ADVERSE REACTIONS AND SIDE EFFECTS

CNS: dizziness, headache.
CV: VENTRICULAR ARRHYTHMIAS, chest pain, QT interval prolongation.

INTERACTIONS

Drug-Drug: ■ Concurrent use of renal cation transport inhibitors including **cimetidine, trimethoprim,** and **ketoconazole** increases blood levels and the risk of serious arrhythmias and is contraindicated ■ **Amiloride, metformin, megestrol, prochlorperazine,** and **triamterene** may have similar effects ■ Blood levels and risk of arrhythmias are also increased by **verapamil**; concurrent use is contraindicated and a 2 day washout-period is recommended) ■ Inhibitors of the cytochrome P450 system (CY P450 3A4 isoenzyme) including **macrolide anti-infectives, azole antifungals, protease inhibitor antiretorivirals, selective serotinin reuptake inhibitor antidepressants, amiodarone, cannabinoids, diltiazem, nefazodone, quinine,** and **zafirlukast** may also increase blood levels and the risk of arrhythmias and should concurrent use be undertaken with caution ■ Should not be used concurrently with other **group I or III antiarrhythmics** due to increased risk of arrhythmias ■ **Bepridil,** some **macrolide anti-infectives, phenothiazines,** and **tricyclic antidepressants** also prolong QT interval and should not be used concurrently with dofetilide ■ Hypokalemia or hypomagnesemia from **potassium-depleting diuretics** increases the risk of arrhythmias; correct abnormalities prior to administration ■ Concurrent use of **digoxin** may also increase the risk of arrhythmias.

ROUTE AND DOSAGE

❑ **Dosing should be adjusted according to renal function and assessment of QT interval.**

■ **PO (Adults):** *Starting dose*—500 mcg twice daily; *maintenace dose*—250 mcg twice daily (not to exceed 500 mcg twice daily).

❑ **Renal Impairment**

■ **PO (Adults):**

■ CCr 40 –60 ml/min

■ *Starting dose*—250 mcg twice daily; *maintenance dose*— 125 mcg twice daily.

■ CCr 20 – 40 ml/min

■ *Starting dose*—125 mcg twice daily; *maintenance dose*—125 mcg once daily.

AVAILABILITY

■ *Capsules:* 125 mcg, 250 mcg, 500 mcg.

TIME/ACTION PROFILE (blood levels)

	ONSET	PEAK	DURATION
PO	within hours	2-3 hr*	12-24 hr

*Steady state levels are achieved after 2–3 days.

NURSING IMPLICATIONS

ASSESSMENT

❑ Monitor ECG, pulse, and blood pressure continuously throughout initiation or therapy and for at least 3 days, then periodically throughout therapy. QTc should be evaluated prior to initiation of therapy and every 3 months throughout therapy. If QTc exceeds 440 msec (500 msec in patients with ventricular conduction abnormalities), dofetilide should be discontinued and patient should be carefully monitored until QTc returns to baseline.

❑ Assess the patient's medication history including OTC, Rx, and herbal/alternative/complementary preparations, with emphasis on those that interact with dofetilide (see Interactions).

■ *Lab Test Considerations:* Creatinine clearance must be calculated for all patients prior to administration and every 3 months throughout therapy.

POTENTIAL NURSING DIAGNOSES

■ Cardiac output, decreased (Indications).
■ Knowledge deficit, related to medication regimen (Patient/Family Teaching).

IMPLEMENTATION

■ **General Info:** Dolfetilide must be initiated or reinitiated in a setting that provides continuous ECG monitoring and has personnel trained in the management of serious ventricular arrhythmias. Due to the potential for life-threatening ventricular arrhythmias, dofetilide is usually used for patients with highly symptomatic AF/AFl.

❑ Patients with AF should be anticoagulated according to usual protocol prior to electrical or pharmacologic cardioversion.

❑ Make sure patient has an adequate supply of dofetilide prior to discharge to prevent interruption of therapy.

❑ Patients should not be discharged from the hospital within 12 hrs of electrical or pharmacologic conversion to normal sinus rhythm.

■ **PO:** Administer at the same time each day without regard to food.

PATIENT/FAMILY TEACHING

❑ Instruct patient to take medication exactly as directed, even if feeling well. If a dose is missed, do not double next dose. Take next dose at usual time.

❑ Patient should read the patient package insert prior to initiation of therapy and reread it each time therapy is renewed. Emphasize the need for compliance with therapy, the potential for drug interactions, and the need for periodic monitoring to minimize the risk of serious arrhythmias.

❑ Instruct patient or family member on how to take pulse. Advise patient to report changes in pulse rate or rhythm to health care professional.

❑ May cause dizziness. Caution patient to avoid driving or other activities requiring alertness until response to medication is known.

❑ Advise patients to inform health care professional of medication regimen prior to treatment or surgery.

❑ Instruct patient not to take OTC medications with dofetilide without consulting health care professional.

❑ Advise patients to consult health care professional immediately if they faint, become dizzy, or have fast heartbeats. If health care professional is unavailable, instruct patient to go to nearest hospital emergency department with the remaining dofetilide capsules, and show them to the doctor or nurse. If symptoms associated with altered electrolyte balance such as excessive or prolonged diarrhea, sweating, vomiting, loss of appetite, or thirst occur, health care professional should also be notified immediately.

❑ Emphasize the importance of routine follow-up exams to monitor progress.

EVALUATION

Clinical response to therapy can be evaluated by:■ Prevention of recurrent AF/AFl ■ Conversion of AF/AFl to normal sinus rhythm ❑ If patients do not convert to normal sinus rhythm within 24 hr of initiation of therapy, electrical conversion should be considered.

EFLORNITHINE
(ee-**flor**-ni-theen)
Vaniqa

CLASSIFICATION(S):
Dermatologic agents (facial hair remover) (topical)

Pregnancy Category C

INDICATIONS

■ Reduction of unwanted facial hair in women.

ACTION

■ Inhibits the enzyme ornithine decarboxylase (ODC) in skin, which decreases synthesis of polyamines. Therapeutic Effects:■ Decreased hair growth in areas of application.

PHARMACOKINETICS

Absorption: Less than 1%.
Distribution: UK.
Metabolism and Excretion: Small amounts absorbed are excreted unchanged in urine.
Half-life: 8 hr.

CONTRAINDICATIONS AND PRECAUTIONS

Contraindicated in: ■ Hypersensitivity.
Use Cautiously in: ■ Pregnancy, lactation or children <12 yr (safety not established).

ADVERSE REACTIONS AND SIDE EFFECTS

Local: burning, rash, stinging, tingling.

INTERACTIONS

Drug-Drug: ■ None known.

ROUTE AND DOSAGE

■ **Topical (Adults):** Apply a thin layer to affected areas of the face and adjacent involved areas under the chin and rub in thoroughly. Do not wash for 4 hours following application. Use twice daily at least 8 hr apart.

AVAILABILITY

■ *13.9 % cream:* 30 g tube.

TIME/ACTION PROFILE (decreased hair growth)

	ONSET	PEAK	DURATION
topical	4–8 wk	UK	8 wk*

*Following discontinuation.

NURSING IMPLICATIONS

ASSESSMENT

❑ Assess facial hair prior to and every few weeks during therapy.

POTENTIAL NURSING DIAGNOSES

■ Risk for impaired skin integrity.

IMPLEMENTATION

■ **Topical:** Apply a thin layer of eflornithine to affected areas of the face and adjacent affected areas under the chin and rub in thoroughly twice daily at least 8 hr apart. Do not wash area for at least 4 hrs.

❑ Avoid getting medication in eyes or inside nose or mouth. If medication gets in eyes, rinse thoroughly with water and notify health care professional.

❑ Hair removal techniques should be continued as needed concurrently with eflornithine.

PATIENT/FAMILY TEACHING

❑ Instruct patient in the correct technique for application of eflornithine. If a dose is missed, do not try to make it up; return to normal application schedule. Advise patient that medication does not permanently remove hair or cure unwanted facial hair. It is not a depilatory. Current hair removal technique should continue. Eflornithine helps manage condition and improve appearance. Hair will return to pretreatment condition in about 8 wks after discontinuation.

❑ Advise patient that normal cosmetics or sunscreen may be used after eflornithine application. Wait a few minutes to allow treatment to be absorbed before applying them.

❑ Inform patient that eflornithine may cause temporary redness, rash, burning, stinging, or tingling, especially when the skin is damaged. Folliculitis or hair bumps may also occur. If irritation continues or condition worsens, stop medication and notify health care professional.

❑ Advise patient to notify health care professional before taking any Rx or OTC medications or using any facial or skin creams.

❑ Advise patient to inform health care professional if pregnancy is planned or suspected or if breast feeding an infant.

EVALUATION

Clinical response to therapy can be evaluated by: ■ Gradual decrease in hair growth in areas of application. Improvement may be seen in 4–8 wks or longer. If no improvement is seen after 6 months of use, discontinue use.

INSULIN ASPART
(in-su-lin as-spart)
NovoLog

CLASSIFICATION(S):
Antidiabetic agents (pancreatic hormone)

Pregnancy Category C

INDICATIONS

■ Control of blood sugar in adult patients with diabetes mellitus.

ACTION

■ Lowers blood glucose by increasing transport into cells and promoting the conversion of glucose to glycogen ■ Promotes the conversion of amino acids to proteins in muscle and stimulates triglyceride formation ■ Inhibits the release of free fatty acids ■ Has a more rapid onset and shorter duration than regular human insulin; should be used with an intermediate- or long-acting insulin. Therapeutic Effects: ■ Control of blood sugar in diabetic patients.

PHARMACOKINETICS

Absorption: Faster absorption, faster onset of action and shorter duration of action than regular human insulin.
Distribution: UK.
Metabolism and Excretion: Insulin is metabolized by liver, spleen, kidney, and muscle.

Half-life: 5–6 min (prolonged in diabetic patients; biologic half-life is longer).

CONTRAINDICATIONS AND PRECAUTIONS

Contraindicated in: ■ Allergy or hypersensitivity to insulin aspart.

Use Cautiously in: ■ Stress, pregnancy, and infection (temporarily increase insulin requirements) ■ Children (safety not established).

ADVERSE REACTIONS AND SIDE EFFECTS

CV: edema.

Derm: urticaria.

Endo: HYPOGLYCEMIA, rebound hyperglycemia (Somogyi effect).

F and E: sodium retention.

Local: lipodystrophy, itching, lipohypertrophy, redness, swelling.

Misc: allergic reactions including ANAPHYLAXIS.

INTERACTIONS

Drug-Drug: ■ **Beta-adrenergic blocking agents**, **clonidine**, **guanethidine**, and **reserpine** may block some of the signs and symptoms of hypoglycemia and delay recovery from hypoglycemia ■ **Thiazide diuretics**, **corticosteroids**, **danazol**, **diltiazem**, **dobutamine**, **thyroid preparations**, **estrogens**, **isoniazid**, **nicotine**, **phenothiazines**, **progesterone**, **protease inhibitor antiretrovirals**, **somatropin**, **thyroid hormones**, **sympathomimetic agents**, and **rifampin** may increase insulin requirements. ■ Anabolic steroids (**testosterone**), **alcohol**, **ACE inhibitors**, **clofibrate**, **disopyramide**, **fluoxetine**, **guanethidine**, **MAO inhibitors**, most **NSAIDs**, **octreotide**, **oral hypoglycemic agents**, **propoxyphene**, **sulfinpyrazone**, **salicylates**, **tetracyclines**, **phenylbutazone**, and **warfarin** may decrease insulin requirements.

ROUTE AND DOSAGE

■ **SC (Adults and Children):** Determined by needs of the patients; generally 0.5–1 units/kg/day. 50–70% may be given as insulin aspart, nd the remainder as intermediate- or long-acting insulin.

AVAILABILITY

■ *Solution for SC injection:* 100 units/ml in 10-ml vials and 3-ml PenFill cartidges for use with NovoPen 3 Insulin Delivery Devices and NovoFine disposable needles.

TIME/ACTION PROFILE (hypoglycemic effect)

	ONSET	PEAK	DURATION
SC	rapid	1–3 hr	3–5 hr

NURSING IMPLICATIONS

ASSESSMENT

❑ Assess patient periodically for symptoms of hypoglycemia (anxiety; chills; cold sweats; confusion; cool, pale skin; difficulty in concentration; drowsiness; excessive hunger; headache; irritability; nausea; nervousness; rapid pulse; shakiness; unusual tiredness or weakness) and hyperglycemia (drowsiness; flushed, dry skin; fruit-like breath odor; frequent urination; loss of appetite; tiredness; unusual thirst) throughout therapy.

❑ Monitor body weight periodically. Changes in weight may necessitate changes in insulin dose.

■ *Lab Test Considerations:* Monitor blood glucose and ketones every 6 hr throughout therapy, more frequently in ketoacidosis and times of stress. Glycosylated hemoglobin may also be monitored to determine effectiveness of therapy.

■ *Toxicity and Overdose:* Overdose is manifested by symptoms of hypoglycemia. Mild hypoglycemia may be treated by ingestion of oral glucose. Severe hypoglycemia is a life-threatening emergency; treatment consists of IV glucose, glucagon, or epinephrine.

POTENTIAL NURSING DIAGNOSES

■ Knowledge deficit, related to medication regimen (Patient/Family Teaching).

■ Noncompliance (Patient/Family Teaching).

IMPLEMENTATION

■ **General Info:** Check type, species source, dose, and expiration date with another licensed nurse. Do not interchange insulins without consulting physician or other health care professional.

□ Use *only* insulin syringes to draw up dose. The unit markings on the insulin syringe must match the insulin's units/ml.

□ When mixing insulins, draw insulin aspart into syringe first to avoid contamination of regular insulin vial. Administer immediately after mixing. Do not mix with crystalline zinc insulin preparations.

□ Insulin aspart should be refrigerated, but do not freeze or administer solution if it has been frozen. Cartridges or vials may be kept at room temperature for up to 28 days if kept from excessive heat and sunlight. Do not use if cloudy, discolored, or unusually viscous.

□ Because of short duration of effects of insulin aspart, supplementation with longer-acting insulin is usually necessary to control blood glucose levels.

■ **SC:** Administer insulin aspart SC in the abdominal wall, thigh, or upper arm within 5–10 min before a meal. Rotate injection sites. Do not administer IV.

PATIENT/FAMILY TEACHING

□ Instruct patient on proper technique for administration. Include type of insulin, equipment (syringe, cartridge pens, alcohol swabs), storage, and place to discard syringes. Discuss the importance of not changing brands of insulin or syringes, selection and rotation of injection sites, and compliance with therapeutic regimen.

□ Demonstrate technique for mixing insulins by drawing up insulin aspart first and rolling intermediate-acting insulin vial between palms to mix, rather than shaking (may cause inaccurate dose).

□ Explain to patient that this medication controls hyperglycemia but does not cure diabetes. Therapy is long term.

□ Instruct patient in proper testing of serum glucose and ketones. These tests should be closely monitored during periods of stress or illness and health care professional notified of significant changes.

□ Emphasize the importance of compliance with nutritional guidelines and regular exercise as directed by health care professional.

□ Advise patient to consult health care professional prior to consuming alcohol or other medications concurrently with insulin.

□ Advise patient to notify health care professional of medication regimen prior to treatment or surgery.

□ Advise patient to notify health care professional if nausea, vomiting, or fever develops, if unable to eat regular diet, or if blood sugar levels are not controlled.

□ Instruct patient on signs and symptoms of hypoglycemia and hyperglycemia and what to do if they occur.

□ Advise patient to notify health care professional if pregnancy is planned or suspected.

□ Patients with diabetes mellitus should carry a source of sugar (candy, sugar packets) and identification describing their disease and treatment regimen at all times.

□ Emphasize the importance of regular follow-up, especially during first few weeks of therapy.

EVALUATION

Effectiveness of therapy can be demonstrated by: ■ Control of blood glucose levels without the appearance of hypoglycemic or hyperglycemic episodes.

INSULIN GLARGINE
(**in**-su-lin **glar**-jeen)
Lantus

CLASSIFICATION(S):
Antidiabetic agents (pancreatic hormone)

Pregnancy Category C

INDICATIONS

■ Indicated for once-daily SC administration at bedtime in the treatment of adult and pediatric patients with type 1 diabetes mellitus or adult patients with type 2 diabetes mellitus who require basal (long-acting) insulin for the control of hyperglycemia.

ACTION

■ Lowers blood glucose by increasing transport into cells and promoting the conversion of glucose to glycogen ■ Promotes the conversion of amino acids to proteins in muscle and stimulate triglyceride formation ■ Inhibits the release of free fatty acids **Therapeutic Effects:** ■ Control of blood sugar in diabetic patients.

PHARMACOKINETICS

Absorption: Provides slower prolonged absorption and a relatively constant concentrations over 24 hr.
Distribution: UK.
Metabolism and Excretion: Partially metabolized at the site of injection to active insulin metabolites. Insulin is metabolized by the liver, the spleen, the kidney, and muscle tissue.
Half-life: 5–6 min (prolonged in diabetic patients; biological half-life is longer).

CONTRAINDICATIONS AND PRECAUTIONS

Contraindicated in: ■ Allergy or hypersensitivity to insulin glargine.
Use Cautiously in: ■ Stress, pregnancy, and infection (may temporarily increase insulin requirements).

ADVERSE REACTIONS AND SIDE EFFECTS

CV: edema.
Derm: rash, urticaria.
Endo: HYPOGLYCEMIA, rebound hyperglycemia (Somogyi effect).
F and E: sodium retention.
Local: lipodystrophy, injection site pain, itching, redness, swelling.
Misc: allergic reactions including ANAPHYLAXIS.

INTERACTIONS

Drug-Drug: ■ **Beta-adrenergic blocking agents, clonidine, guanethidine,** and **reserpine** may block some of the signs and symptoms of hypoglycemia and delay recovery from hypoglycemia ■ **Thiazide diuretics, corticosteroids, danazol, diltiazem, dobutamine, thyroid preparations, estrogens, isoniazid, nicotine, phenothiazines, progesterone, protease inhibitors, antiretrovirals, somatropin, thyroid hormones, sympathomimetic agents,** and **rifampin** may increase insulin requirements ■ Anabolic steroids (**testosterone**), **alcohol, ACE inhibitors, clofibrate, disopyramide, fluoxetine, guanethidine, MAO in-**

hibitors, most **NSAIDs, octreotide, oral hypoglycemic agents, propoxyphene, sulfinpyrazone, salicylates, tetracyclines, phenylbutazone,** and **warfarin** may decrease insulin requirements.

ROUTE AND DOSAGE

■ **SC (Adults and Children ≥6 yr):** *Initiation in patients with type 2 diabetes already being treated with oral antidiabetic agents*—10 units once daily; then adjusted on the basis of patient's needs (range 2–100 units/day); *Change over from other intermediate- or long-acting insulin.* Decrease total daily NPH dose by 20% during the first week, then adjust on the basis of patient's needs.

AVAILABILITY

■ *Solution for SC injection:* 100 units/ml in 5-ml vials, 10 ml-vials, and 3-ml cartidges for use with OptiPen One Insulin Delivery Device.

TIME/ACTION PROFILE (hypoglycemic effect)

	ONSET	PEAK	DURATION
SC	within 1 hr	5 hr	24 hr

NURSING IMPLICATIONS

ASSESSMENT

❑ Assess patient for signs and symptoms of hypoglycemia (anxiety; chills; cold sweats; confusion; cool, pale skin; difficulty in concentration; drowsiness; excessive hunger; headache; irritability; nausea; nervousness; rapid pulse; shakiness; unusual tiredness or weakness) and hyperglycemia (drowsiness; flushed, dry skin; fruit-like breath odor; frequent urination; loss of appetite; tiredness; unusual thirst) periodically throughout therapy.

❑ Monitor body weight periodically. Changes in weight may necessitate changes in insulin dose.

■ *Lab Test Considerations:*

❑ Monitor blood glucose and ketones every 6 hr throughout therapy, more frequently in ketoacidosis and times of stress. Glycosylated hemoglobin may also be monitored to determine effectiveness of therapy.

■ *Toxicity and Overdose:* Overdose is manifested by symptoms of hypoglycemia. Mild hypoglycemia may be treated by ingestion of oral glucose. Severe hypoglycemia is a life-threatening emergency; treatment consists of IV glucose, glucagon, or epinephrine. Recovery from hypoglycemia may be delayed due to the prolonged effect of SC insulin glargine.

POTENTIAL NURSING DIAGNOSES

■ Knowledge deficit, related to medication regimen (Patient/Family Teaching).
■ Noncompliance (Patient/Family Teaching).

IMPLEMENTATION

■ **General Info:** When transferring from once-daily NPH human insulin or ultralente insulin to insulin glargine, the dosage usually remains unchanged. When transferring from twice-daily NPH human insulin to insulin glargine, the initial dose of insulin glargine is usually reduced by 20%.
❑ Do not mix insulin glargine with any other insulin or solution, or use syringes containing any other medicinal product or residue. Solution should be clear and colorless with no particulate matter.
❑ Use *only* insulin syringes to draw up dose. Insulin syringe or OptiPen One can be used for administration. Prior to withdrawing dose, rotate vial between palms to ensure uniform solution; do not shake.
❑ Store unopened vials and cartridges in the refrigerator; do not freeze. If unable to refrigerate, the 10-ml vial can be kept in a cool place unrefrigerated for up to 28 days, and the 5-ml vial, up to 14 days. Once the cartridge is placed in an OptiPen One, do not refrigerate.
■ **SC:** Administer SC once daily at bedtime. Do not administer IV.

PATIENT/FAMILY TEACHING

❑ Instruct patient on proper technique for administration. Include type of insulin, equipment (syringe, cartridge pens, alcohol swabs), storage, and place to discard syringes. Discuss the importance of selection and rotation of injection sites, and compliance with therapeutic regimen.

❑ Explain to patient that this medication controls hyperglycemia but does not cure diabetes. Therapy is long term.
❑ Instruct patient in proper testing of serum glucose and ketones. These tests should be closely monitored during periods of stress or illness and health care professional notified of significant changes.
❑ Emphasize the importance of compliance with nutritional guidelines and regular exercise, as directed by health care professional.
❑ Advise patient to consult health care professional prior to consuming alcohol or other medications concurrently with insulin.
❑ Advise patient to notify health care professional of medication regimen prior to treatment or surgery.
❑ Advise patient to notify health care professional if nausea, vomiting, or fever develops, if unable to eat regular diet, or if blood sugar levels are not controlled.
❑ Instruct patient on signs and symptoms of hypoglycemia and hyperglycemia and on what to do if they occur.
❑ Advise patient to notify health care professional if pregnancy is planned or suspected.
❑ Patients with diabetes mellitus should carry a source of sugar (candy, sugar packets) and identification describing their disease and treatment regimen at all times.
❑ Emphasize the importance of regular follow-up, especially during first few weeks of therapy.

EVALUATION

Effectiveness of therapy can be demonstrated by: ■ Control of blood glucose levels without the appearance of hypoglycemic or hyperglycemic episodes.

LINEZOLID
(li-**nez**-o-lid)
Zyvox

CLASSIFICATION(S):
Anti-infective agents (oxazolidinone)

Pregnancy Category C

INDICATIONS

■ Treatment of the following infections: ❑ Infections caused by vancomycin-resistant *Enterococcus faecium* ❑ Nosocomial pneumonia caused by *Staphylococcus aureus* (methicillin-susceptible and -resistant strains) ❑ Complicated skin/skin structure infections caused by *Staphylococcus aureus* (methicillin-susceptible and -resistant strains), *Streptococcus pyogenes* or *Streptococcus agalactiae* ❑ Uncomplicated skin/skin structure infections caused by *Staphylococcus aureus* (methicillin-susceptible and -resistant strains), *Streptococcus pyogenes* ❑ Community-acquired pneumonia caused by *Streptococcus pneumoniae* (penicillin-susceptible strains only) or *Staphylococcus aureus* (methicillin-susceptible strains only).

ACTION

■ Inhibits bacterial protein synthesis at the level of the 23S ribosome of the 50S subunit. Therapeutic Effects: ■ Bactericidal action against streptococci; bacteriostatic action against enterococci and staphylococci.

PHARMACOKINETICS

Absorption: Rapidly and extensively (100%) absorbed following oral administration.
Distribution: Readily distributes to well-perfused tissues.
Metabolism and Excretion: 65 % metabolized, mostly by the liver; 30% excreted unchanged by the kidneys.
Half-life: 6.4 hr.

CONTRAINDICATIONS AND PRECAUTIONS

Contraindicated in: ■ Hypersensitivity ■ Phenylketonuria (suspension contains aspartame).
Use Cautiously in: ■ Thrombocytopenia, concurrent use of antiplatelet agents or bleeding diathesis (platelet counts should be monitored more frequently) ■ Pregnancy, lactation or children (safety not established).

ADVERSE REACTIONS AND SIDE EFFECTS

CV: headache, insomnia.
GI: PSEUDOMEMBRANOUS COLITIS, diarrhea, increased liver function tests, nausea, taste alteration, vomiting.

Hemat: thrombocytopenia.

INTERACTIONS

Drug-Drug: ■ Linezolid has monoamine oxidase inhibitory properties; response to **indirect-acting sympathomimetics**, **vasopressors**, or **dopaminergic agents** may be enhanced. Initial doses of **adrenergic agents** such as **dopamine** or **epinephrine** should be reduced and carefully titrated.
Drug-Food: ■ Because of monoamine oxidase inhibitory properties, consumption of large amounts of foods or beverages containing tyramine should be avoided, due to risk of increased pressor response (See Appendix L of Davis's Drug Guide for Nurses, ed 7.)

ROUTE AND DOSAGE

❑ **Vancomycin-resistant *Enterococcus faecium* infections**
■ **PO, IV (Adults):** 600 mg q 12 hr for 14–28 days.

❑ **Pneumonia, complicated skin/skin structure infections**
■ **PO, IV (Adults):** 600 mg q 12 hr for 10–14 days.

❑ **Uncomplicated skin/skin structure infections**
■ **PO (Adults):** 400 mg q 12 hr for 10–14 days.

AVAILABILITY

■ *Oral suspension: (orange):* 100 mg/5 ml^{Rx}
■ *Tablets:* 400 mg^{Rx}, 600 mg^{Rx} ■ *Solution for injection:* 200 mg/100 ml bag, 400 mg/200 ml bag and 600 mg/300 ml bag^{Rx}

TIME/ACTION PROFILE

	ONSET	PEAK	DURATION
PO	rapid	1–2 hr	12 hr
IV	rapid	end of infusion	12 hr

NURSING IMPLICATIONS

ASSESSMENT

■ **General Info:** Assess patient for infection (vital signs; appearance of wound, sputum, urine, and stool; WBC) at beginning of and throughout therapy.

□ Obtain specimens for culture and sensitivity prior to initiating therapy. First dose may be given before receiving results.

■ **Pseudomembranous Colitis:** Assess bowel status (bowel sounds, frequency and consistency of stools, presence of blood in stools) throughout therapy.

■ *Lab Test Considerations:* May cause thrombocytopenia. Monitor platelet count in patients who are at risk for increased bleeding, who have pre-existing thrombocytopenia, who receive concurrent medications that may decrease platelet count, or who may require >2 weeks of therapy.

□ May cause increased AST, ALT, LDH, alkaline phosphatase, and BUN.

POTENTIAL NURSING DIAGNOSES

■ Infection, risk for (Indications).

■ Knowledge deficit, related to medication regimen (Patient/Family Teaching).

IMPLEMENTATION

■ **General Info:** Dosage adjustment is not necessary when switching from IV to oral dose.

■ **PO:** May be administered with or without food.

□ Before using gently invert 3–5 times to mix; do not shake. Store at room temperature.

■ **Intermittent Infusion:** Injection is administered in single- and ready-to-use infusion bags. Do not administer infusion containing particulate matter.

■ *Rate:* Administer over 30–120 minutes. Do not use bag in series connections. Flush line before and after infusion.

■ **Y-Site Compatibility:** ■ D5W ■ 0.9% NaCl ■ lactated Ringer's injection.

■ **Y-Site Incompatibility:**

□ amphotericin B

□ ceftriaxone

□ chlorpromazine

□ diazepam

□ erythromycin lactobionate

□ pentamidine

□ phenytoin

□ trimethoprim/sulfamethoxazole.

PATIENT/FAMILY TEACHING

□ Advise patients taking oral linezolid to take exactly as directed. Tell patients that missed doses should be taken as soon as remembered unless almost time for next dose; do not double dose.

□ Instruct patient to avoid large quantities of foods or beverages containing tyramine (See Appendix L of *Davis's Drug Guide for Nurses*, ed 7). May cause hypertensive response.

□ Instruct patient to notify health care professional if patient has a history of hypertension and before patient takes other medications, especially cold remedies, decongestants, or antidepressants.

□ Advise patient to notify health care professional if no improvement is seen in a few days.

EVALUATION

Clinical response to therapy can be evaluated by: ■ Resolution of signs and symptoms of infection. Length of time for complete resolution depends on organism and site of infection.

LOPINAVIR/RITONAVIR
(loe-**pin**-a-veer/ri-**toe**-na-veer)
Kaletra

CLASSIFICATION(S):
Antiretroviral agents (protease inhibitor)

Pregnancy Category C

INDICATIONS

■ Management of HIV infection in combination with other antiretrovirals.

ACTION

■ **Lopinavir:** Inhibits HIV viral protease. ■ **Ritonavir:** Although ritonavir has antiretroviral activity of its own (inhibits the action of HIV protease and prevents the cleavage of viral polyproteins), it is combined with lopinavir to inhibit the metabolism of lopinavir thus increasing its plasma levels. Therapeutic Effects: ■ Increased CD4 cell counts and decreased viral load with subsequent slowed progression of HIV infection and its sequelae.

PHARMACOKINETICS

Absorption: Appears to be well absorbed following oral administration; food enhances absorption.

Distribution: *Ritonavir*—poor CNS penetration.

Protein Binding: *Lopinavir*—98–99% bound to plasma proteins.

Metabolism and Excretion: *Lopinavir*—completely metabolized in the liver by cytochrome P450 P3A (CY P450 P3A); ritonavir is a potent inhibitor of this enzyme. *Ritonavir*—highly metabolized by the liver (by CY P450 P3A and CY P2D6 enzymes); one metabolite has antiretroviral activity; 3.5% excreted unchanged in urine.

Half-life: *Lopinavir*—5–6 hr; *Ritonavir*—3–5 hr.

CONTRAINDICATIONS AND PRECAUTIONS

Contraindicated in: ■ Hypersensitivity ■ Concurrent use of the following agents, which are highly dependent on CY P450 P3A or CY P2D6 for metabolism and for which increased blood levels may result in serious and/or life-threatening events including: dihydroergotamine, ergotamine, ergonovine, flecainide, methylergonovine, midazolam, pimozide, propafenone, and triazolam ■ Concurrent use with simastatin, lovastatin, St. John's wort (*Hypericum perforatum*) is not recommended ■ Hypersensitivity or intolerance to alcohol or castor oil (present in capsules and liquid).

Use Cautiously in: ■ Known alcohol intolerance (oral solution contains alcohol) ■ Concurrent use with atorvastatin or cerivastatin (may increase risk of rhabdomyolysis) ■ Concurrent use of antiarrhythmics including amiodarone, bepridil, lidocaine, and quinidine (therapeutic blood level monitoring recommended) ■ Concurrent use of anticonvulsants including carbamazepine, phenobarbital or phenytoin (may decrease effectiveness of lopinavir) ■ Concurrent use of dihydropyridine calcium channel blockers including felodipine, nifedipine, and nicardipine (clinical monitoring recommended due to increased levels of calcium channel blocker) ■ Impaired hepatic function, history of hepatitis (for ritonavir content) ■ Pregnancy or lactation (safety not established; breast feeding not recommended in HIV-infected patients).

Exercise Extreme Caution in: ■ Concurrent use with sildenafil should be undertaken with extreme caution and may result in hypotension, syncope, visual changes, and prolonged erection.

ADVERSE REACTIONS AND SIDE EFFECTS

CNS: headache, insomnia, weakness.
GI: diarrhea, abdominal pain, nausea, pancreatitis, vomiting.
Derm: rash.

INTERACTIONS

Drug-Drug: ■ Concurrent use of flecainide, propafenone, dihydroergotamine, ergonovine, ergotamine, methylergonovine, cisapride, pimozide, midazolam, and triazolam, is contraindicated because of the risk of potentially serious, life-threatening drug interactions. ■ Concurrent use with **rifampin** will decrease effectiveness of antiretroviral therapy and should not be undertaken ■ Should not be used concurrently with **simvastatin** or **lovastatin** due to increased risk of rhabdomyolysis; similar risk exists for **atorvastatin** and **cerivastatin**, use lowest possible dose with careful monitoring ■ Concurrent use with **efavirenz** or **nevirapine** decreases lopinavir/ritonavir levels and effectiveness; dosage increase may be necessary ■ **Delavirdine** increases lopinavir levels ■ Concurrent use of antiarrhythmics including **amiodarone**, **bepridil**, **lidocaine**, and **quinidine** (therapeutic blood level monitoring recommended due to increased levels of antiarrhythmics) ■ Concurrent use of anticonvulsants including **carbamazepine**, **phenobarbital**, or **phenytoin** (may decrease effectiveness of lopinavir) ■ Concurrent use of dihydropyridine calcium channel blockers including **felodipine**, **nifedipine**, and **nicardipine** (clinical monitoring recommended due to increased levels of calcium channel blockers) ■ May alter levels and effectiveness of **warfarin** ■ Increases levels of **clarithromycin** (dosage reduction recommended for patients with CCr ≤60 ml/min ■ Increases blood levels of **itraconazole** and **ketoconazole** (high doses of these antifungals not recommended) ■ Increases levels of **rifabutin** (dosage reduction recommended). ■ Decreases blood levels of **atovaquone** (may require dosage increase) ■ **Dexamethasone** deceases blood levels and may decrease effectiveness of lopinavir ■ Oral solution contains alcohol may produce intolerance when administered with **disulfiram** or **metronidazole** ■ Concurrent use with **sildenafil** should be undertaken with extreme caution and may result in hypotension, syncope, visual changes, and prolonged erection (dosage reduction of sildenafil to 25 mg every 48 hr with monitoring recommended) ■ May increase levels and risk of toxicity with immunosuppressant including **cyclosporine** or **tacrolimus** (blood level monitoring recommended) ■ May decrease blood levels and effects of methadone (dosage of methadone may need to be increased) ■ May decrease levels and contraceptive efficacy of some estrogen-based oral contraceptives including **ethinyl estradiol** (alternative or additional methods of contraception should be used)

Drug-Natural Products: ■ Concurrent use with **St. John's wort (H. perforatum)** may decrease levels and beneficial effect of lopinavir/ritonavir.

ROUTE AND DOSAGE

- **PO (Adults and Children >40 kg):** 400/100 mg (3 capsules or 5 ml oral solution) twice daily.
- **PO (Children 6 mos–12 yr):** 230/57.5 mg/m² twice daily.
- **PO (Children 15–40 kg):** 10 mg/kg lopinavir content twice daily.
- **PO (Children 7<15 kg):** 12 mg/kg lopinavir content twice daily.

❏ **With concurrent efavirenz or nevirapine**

- **PO (Adults and Children >50 mg):** 533/133 mg (4 capsules or 6.5 ml oral solution) twice daily.
- **PO (Children 6 mos–12 yr):** 300/75 mg/m² twice daily.
- **PO (Children 15–50 kg):** 11/2.75 mg/kg twice daily.
- **PO (Children 7–<15 kg):** 13/3.25 mg/kg twice daily.

AVAILABILITY

■ **Capsules:** 133.3 mg lopinavir/33 mg ritonavir ■ **Oral solution:** 80 mg lopinavir/ 20 mg ritonavir per ml (contains 42.4% alcohol).

TIME/ACTION PROFILE (blood levels)

	ONSET	PEAK	DURATION
Lopinavir PO	rapid	4 hr	12 hr
Ritonavir PO	rapid	4 hr*	12 hr

*Non-fasting.

NURSING IMPLICATIONS

ASSESSMENT

❏ Assess patient for change in severity of HIV symptoms and for symptoms of opportunistic infections throughout therapy.

❏ Assess patient for signs of pancreatitis (nausea, vomiting, abdominal pain, increased serum lipase or amylase) periodically throughout therapy. May require discontinuation of therapy.

■ *Lab Test Considerations:* Monitor viral load and CD4 counts regularly during therapy.

❏ Monitor triglyceride and cholesterol levels prior to initiating therapy and periodically during therapy.

❏ May cause hyperglycemia.

❏ May cause elevated serum AST, ALT, GGT, and total bilirubin concentrations.

POTENTIAL NURSING DIAGNOSES

■ Infection, high risk for (Indications).

■ Knowledge deficit, related to disease processes and medication regimen (Patient/Family Teaching).

■ Noncompliance (Patient/Family Teaching).

IMPLEMENTATION

■ **General Info:** Do not confuse with Retrovir (zidovudine) or ritonavir (Norvir).

❏ Patients taking concurrent didanosine should take didanosine 1 hr before or 2 hr after taking lopinavir/ritonavir.

■ **PO:** Administer with food to enhance absorption.

❏ Oral solution is light yellow to orange.

❏ Capsules and oral solution are stable if refrigerated until expiration date on label or 2 months at room temperature.

PATIENT/FAMILY TEACHING

❏ Emphasize the importance of taking lopinavir/

ritonavir exactly as directed, at evenly spaced times throughout day. Do not take more than prescribed amount, and do not stop taking this or other antiretrovirals without consulting health care professional. If a dose is missed, take as soon as remembered; do not double doses.

❏ Instruct patient that lopinavir/ritonavir should not be shared with others.

❏ Advise patient to avoid taking other medications, Rx, OTC, or herbal alternative, especially St. John's wort, without consulting health care professional.

❏ Inform patient that ritonavir does not cure AIDS or prevent associated or opportunistic infections. Ritonavir does not reduce the risk of transmission of HIV to others through sexual contact or blood contamination. Caution patient to use a condom during sexual contact and to avoid sharing needles or donating blood to prevent spreading the AIDS virus to others. Advise patient that the long-term effects of ritonavir are unknown at this time.

❏ Inform patient that lopinavir/ritonavir may cause hyperglycemia. Advise patient to notify health care professional if increased thirst or hunger, unexplained weight loss, or increased urination occurs.

❏ Advise patients taking oral contraceptives to use a nonhormonal method of birth control during lopinavir/ritonavir therapy.

❏ Caution patients taking sildenafil of increased risk of sildenafil-associated side effects (hypotension, visual changes, sustained erection). Notify health care professional promptly if these occur.

❏ Inform patient that redistribution and accumulation of body fat may occur causing central obesity, dorsocervical fat enlargement (buffalo hump), peripheral wasting, breast enlargement, and cushingoid appearance. The cause and long-term effects are not known.

❏ Instruct patient to notify health care professional if pregnancy is planned or suspected of if breastfeeding an infant.

❏ Emphasize the importance of regular follow-up exams and blood counts to determine progress and monitor for side effects.

EVALUATION

Effectiveness of therapy can be demonstrated by: ■ Delayed progression of AIDS and decreased opportunistic infections in patients with HIV ■ Decrease in viral load and improvement in CD4 cell counts.

MELOXICAM
(me-**lox**-i-kam)
Mobic

CLASSIFICATION(S):
Nonsteroidal anti-inflammatory agents

Pregnancy Category C

INDICATIONS

■ Relief of signs and symptoms of osteoarthritis.

ACTION

■ Inhibit prostaglandin synthesis, probably by inhibiting the enzyme cyclooxygenase. Therapeutic Effects: ■ Decreased pain and inflammation associated with osteoarthritis ■ Also decreases fever.

PHARMACOKINETICS

Absorption: Well absorbed following oral administration.
Distribution: Unknown.
Protein Binding: 99.4%.
Metabolism and Excretion: Mostly metabolized to inactive metabolites by the liver via the P450 enzyme system; metabolites are exreted in urine and feces.
Half-life: 20.1 hr.

CONTRAINDICATIONS AND PRECAUTIONS

Contraindicated in: ■ Hypersensitivity ■ Cross sensitivity may occur with other NSAIDs, including aspirin ■ Severe renal impairment (CCr ≤15 ml/min) ■ Concurrent use of aspirin (increased risk of adverse reactions).

Use Cautiously in: ■ Dehydration (correct deficits before inititating therapy) ■ Impaired renal function, heart failure, liver dysfunction, geriatric patients (≥65 yr), concurrent ACE inhibitor or diuretic therapy (increased risk of reversible renal dysfunction) ■ Coagulation disorders or concurrent anticoagulant therapy (may increase risk of bleeding) ■ Pregnancy, lactation or children <18 yr (safety not established; avoid use late in pregnancy).

ADVERSE REACTIONS AND SIDE EFFECTS

CV: edema.
GI: GI BLEEDING, abnormal liver function tests, diarrhea, dyspepsia, nausea.
Derm: pruritus.
Hemat: anemia, leukopenia, thrombocytopenia.

INTERACTIONS

Drug-Drug: ■ May decrease the antihypertensive effects of **ACE inhibitors** ■ May decrease the diuretic effects of **furosemide** or **thiazide diuretics** ■ Concurrent use with **aspirin** increases meloxicam blood levels and may increase risk of adverse reactions ■ Concurrent use with **cholestyramine** decreases blood levels ■ Increases plasma **lithium** levels (close monitoring recommended when meloxicam is introduced or withdrawn) ■ May increase the risk of bleeding with **anticoagulants**, including **warfarin**.

ROUTE AND DOSAGE

■ **PO (Adults):** 7.5 mg once daily; some patients may require 15 mg/day.

AVAILABILITY

■ **Tablets:** 7.5 mg.

TIME/ACTION PROFILE

	ONSET	PEAK*	DURATION
PO	unk	4.9 hr	24 hr

*Blood levels.

NURSING IMPLICATIONS

ASSESSMENT

■ **General Info:** Patients who have asthma, aspirin-induced allergy, and nasal polyps are at increased risk for developing hypersensitivity reactions. Assess for rhinitis, asthma, and urticaria.

■ **General Info:** Assess pain and range of motion prior to and 1–2 hr following administration.

■ *Lab Test Considerations:* BUN, serum creatinine, CBC, and liver function tests should be evaluated periodically in patients receiving prolonged courses of therapy. May cause anemia, thrombocytopenia, leukopenia, and abnormal liver or renal function tests.
❏ Bleeding time may be prolonged.

POTENTIAL NURSING DIAGNOSES

■ Pain (Indications).
■ Impaired physical mobility (Indications).
■ Knowledge deficit, related to medication regimen (Patient/Family Teaching).

IMPLEMENTATION

■ **General Info:** Administration in higher than recommended doses does not provide increased effectiveness but may cause increased side effects.
■ **PO:** May be administered without regard to food.

PATIENT/FAMILY TEACHING

❏ Advise patient to take this medication with a full glass of water and to remain in an upright position for 15–30 min after administration.
❏ Instruct patient to take medication exactly as directed. If a dose is missed, it should be taken as soon as remembered but not if almost time for the next dose. Do not double doses.
❏ Caution patient to avoid the concurrent use of alcohol, aspirin, acetaminophen, or other OTC medications without consulting health care professional.
❏ Advise patient to inform health care professional of medication regimen prior to treatment or surgery.
❏ Advise patient to consult health care professional if rash, itching, visual disturbances, weight gain, edema, black stools, or signs of hepatotoxicity (nausea, fatigue, lethargy, jaundice, upper right quadrant tenderness, flu-like symptoms) occur.

EVALUATION

Effectiveness of therapy can be demonstrated by: ■ Relief of pain ■ Improved joint mobility. Patients who do not respond to one NSAID may respond to another.

MIFEPRISTONE
(mi-fe-**priss**-tone)
Mifeprex

CLASSIFICATION(S):
Agents used during pregnancy and lactation(abortifacients) (antiprogestational agent)

Pregnancy Category UK

INDICATIONS

■ Medical termination of intrauterine pregnancy through 49 days' pregnancy.

ACTION

■ Antagonizes endometrial and myometrial effects of progesterone ■ Sensitizes the myometrium to contraction-inducing activity of prostaglandins. Therapeutic Effects: ■ Termination of pregnancy.

PHARMACOKINETICS

Absorption: Rapidly absorbed following oral administration (69% bioavailability).
Distribution: UK.
Protein Binding: 98%.
Metabolism and Excretion: Mostly metabolized by the liver (cytochrome CYP450 3A4 [CYP450 3A4] enzyme system).
Half-life: 18 hr.

CONTRAINDICATIONS AND PRECAUTIONS

Contraindicated in: ■ Presence of an intrauterine device (IUD) ■ Confirmed or suspected ectopic pregnancy ■ Undiagnosed adnexal mass ■ Chronic adrenal failure ■ Concurrent long-term corticosteroid therapy ■ Bleeding disorders or concurrent anticoagulant therapy ■ Inherited porphyrias.
Use Cautiously in: ■ Chronic medical conditions such as cardiovascular, hypertensive, hepatic, renal, or respiratory disease (safety and efficacy not established) ■ Women >35 yrs old or who smoke ≥10 cigarettes/day.

ADVERSE REACTIONS AND SIDE EFFECTS

CNS: dizziness, fainting, headache, weakness.
GI: <u>abdominal pain</u>, <u>diarrhea</u>, <u>nausea</u>, <u>vomiting</u>.
GU: <u>uterine bleeding</u>, <u>uterine cramping</u>, pelvic pain.

INTERACTIONS

Drug-Drug: ■ Blood levels and therapeutic effectiveness may be increased by **ketoconazole**, **itraconazole**, and **erythromycin** ■ Blood levels and effects may be decreased by **rifampin**, **dexamethasone**, **phenytoin**, **phenobarbital**, and **carbamazepine** ■ Mifepristone may decrease metabolism and increase effects of other **drugs metabolized by the CYP 450 3A4 enzyme system**, including **some agents used during general anesthesia**.
Drug-Natural Products: ■ Blood levels and effects may be decreased by **St. John's wort**.
Drug-Food: ■ Blood levels and effects may be increased by **grapefruit juice**.

ROUTE AND DOSAGE

■ **PO (Adults):** *Day 1*—600 mg (given as three 200 mg tablets) as a single dose, followed on *day 3* by 400 mcg misoprostol (Cytotec), unless abortion has occurred and has been confirmed by clinical or ultrasonographic examination (see misoprostol monograph in *Davis's Drug Guide for Nurses*, ed 7, p. 655).

AVAILABILITY

■ *Tablets:* 200 mg.

TIME/ACTION PROFILE (termination of pregnancy)

	ONSET	PEAK	DURATION
PO	UK	within 2 days	UK

NURSING IMPLICATIONS

ASSESSMENT

❑ Determine duration of pregnancy. Pregnancy is dated from the first day of the last menstrual period in a presumed 28-day cycle with ovulation occuring at mid-cycle and can be determined by menstrual history and clinical examination; use ultrasound if duration is uncertain or if ectopic pregnancy is suspected.

❑ Assess amount of bleeding and cramping throughout treatment. Determine if termination is complete on day 14.

▪ *Lab Test Considerations:* Decrease in hemoglobin, hematocrit, and red blood cell counts may occur in women who bleed heavily.

❑ Changes in quantitative human chorionic gonadotropin (hCG) levels are not accurate until at least 10 days after mifepristone administration; complete termination of pregnancy must be confirmed by clinical examination.

POTENTIAL NURSING DIAGNOSES

▪ Pain (Side Effects).

▪ Knowledge deficit, related to medication regimen (Patient/Family Teaching).

IMPLEMENTATION

▪ **General Info:** Mifepristone should be administered only by health care professionals who have read and understood the prescribing information, are able to assess gestational age of an embryo and disgnose ectopic pregnancies, and who are able to provide surgical intervention in cases of incomplete abortion or severe bleeding.

❑ Any IUD should be removed prior to mifepristone adminstration.

❑ Measures to prevent rhesus immunization, similar to those of surgical abortion, should be taken.

▪ **PO:** On *day 1*, after the patient has read the Medication Guide and signed the Patient Agreement, administer three 200/mg tablets as a single dose. On *day 3*, unless abortion has occurred and been confirmed by clinical examination or ultrasound, administer two 200-mcg tablets of misoprostol. On *day 14*, confirm that termination of pregnancy has occurred by clinical examination or ultrasound.

PATIENT/FAMILY TEACHING

❑ Advise patient of the treatment and its effects. Patients must be given a copy of the Medication Guide and Patient Agreement. Patient must understand the necessity of completing the treatment schedule of three office visits (day 1, day 3, and day 14).

❑ Inform patient that vaginal bleeding and uterine cramping will probably occur and that prolonged or heavy vaginal bleeding is not proof of complete expulsion. Bleeding or spotting occurs for an average of 9–16 days; but may continue for more than 30 days. Advise patient that if the treatment fails, there is a risk of fetal malformation; medical abortion failures are managed by surgical termination.

❑ Instruct patient in the steps to take in an emergency situation, including precise instructions and a telephone number to call if she has problems or concerns.

❑ May cause dizziness or fainting. Caution patient not to avoid driving or other activities requiring alertness until response to medication is known.

❑ Caution patient that pregnancy can occur following termination of pregnancy and before resumption of normal menses. Contraception can be initiated as soon as pregnancy termination is confirmed, or before sexual intercourse is resumed.

❑ Advise patient to notify health care professioal if she smokes at least 10 cigarettes a day.

EVALUATION

Clinical response to therapy can be evaluated by: ▪ Termination of an intrauterine pregnancy of less than 49 days duration.

RIVASTIGMINE
(rye-va-**stig**-meen)
Exelon

CLASSIFICATION(S):
Cholineric agents (cholinesterase inhibitor), Anti-Alzheimer's agent

Pregnancy Category B

INDICATIONS

▪ Managment of mild-to-moderate dementia associated with Alzheimer's disease.

ACTION

▪ Enhances cholinergic function by reversible inhibition of cholinesterase ■ Does not alter the course of the disease. Therapeutic Effects: ■ Decreased dementia (temporary) associated with Alzheimer's disease.

PHARMACOKINETICS

Absorption: Well absorbed following oral administration.

Distribution: Widely distributed.

Metabolism and Excretion: Rapidly and extensively metabolized by the liver; metabolites are excreted by the kidneys.

Half-life: 1.5 hr.

CONTRAINDICATIONS AND PRECAUTIONS

Contraindicated in: ■ Hypersensitivity to rivastigmine or other carbamates.

Use Cautiously in: ■ History of asthma or obstructive pulmonary disease ■ History of GI bleeding ■ Sick sinus syndrome or other supraventricular cardiac conduction abnormalities ■ Pregnancy, lactation, or children (safety not established).

ADVERSE REACTIONS AND SIDE EFFECTS

CNS: <u>weakness</u>, dizziness, drowsiness, headache.

CV: edema, heart failure, hypotension.

GI: <u>anorexia</u>, dyspepsia, <u>nausea</u>, <u>vomiting</u>, abdominal pain, flatulence.

Neuro: tremor.

Misc: fever, weight loss.

INTERACTIONS

Drug-Drug: ■ **Nicotine** use may increase metabolism and decrease blood levels.

ROUTE AND DOSAGE

■ **PO (Adults):** 1.5 mg twice daily initially; after at least 2 weeks, dose may be increased to 3 mg twice daily. Further increments may be made at 2-week intervals up to 6 mg twice daily.

AVAILABILITY

■ *Capsules:* 1.5 m, 3 mg, 4.5 mg, 6 mg.
■ *Oral Solution:* 2 mg/ml in 120 ml bottle.

TIME/ACTION PROFILE (improvement in dementia)

	ONSET	PEAK	DURATION
PO	within 2 wk	up to 12 wk	unknown

NURSING IMPLICATIONS

ASSESSMENT

❑ Assess cognitive function (memory, attention, reasoning, language, ability to perform simple tasks) periodically throughout therapy.
❑ Monitor patient for nausea, vomiting, anorexia, and weight loss. Notify health care professional if these side effects occur.

POTENTIAL NURSING DIAGNOSES

■ Thought processes, altered (Indications).
■ Nutrition: altered, less than body requirements (Side Effects).
■ Knowledge deficit (Patient/Family Teaching).

IMPLEMENTATION

■ **General Info:** Rivastigmine oral solution and capsules may be interchanged at equal doses.
■ **PO:** Administer in the morning and evening with food.
❑ Oral solution may be administered directly from syringe provided or mixed with a small glass of water, cold fruit juice, or soda. Mixture should be stirred prior to drinking. Ensure patient drinks entire mixture. Oral solution is stable for 4 hours at room temperature when mixed with cold fruit juice or soda. Do not mix with other solutions.

PATIENT/FAMILY TEACHING

❑ Emphasize the importance of taking rivastigmine at regular intervals as directed.
❑ Explain to patient and caregiver how to use oral dosing syringe provided with oral solution. Remove syringe from protective case and push down and twist child resistant closure to open bottle. Insert syringe into opening in white stopper in bottle. Hold the syringe and pull plunger to the level corresponding to the prescribed dose. Before removing syringe from bottle, push out larger bubbles (small bubbles will not alter dose) by moving plunger up and down a few times. After large bubbles are gone, move plunger to level of dose. Remove syringe from bottle.

- Caution patient and caregiver that rivastigmine may cause dizziness.
- Advise patient and caregiver to notify health care professional if nausea, vomiting, anorexia, or weight loss occur.
- Advise patient and caregiver to notify health care professional of medication regimen prior to treatment or surgery.

EVALUATION

Clinical response to therapy can be evaluated by: ■ Temporary improvement in cognitive function (memory, attention, reasoning, language, ability to perform simple tasks) in patients with Alzheimer's disease.

SAMe
(sam-ee)
Ademetionine, S-adenosylmethionine

CLASSIFICATION(S):
Antidepressants

Pregnancy Category UK

INDICATIONS

■ Treatment of depression ■ Has also been used to manage: ❏ osteoarthritis ❏ fibromyalgia ❏ liver disease ❏ migraine headaches.

ACTION

■ May aid in the production of various amines. Therapeutic Effects: ■ Decreased depression.

PHARMACOKINETICS

Absorption: Rapidly and extensively metabolized following oral administration.
Distribution: Unknown.
Metabolism and Excretion: Actively metabolized by the liver.
Half-life: 80 min.

CONTRAINDICATIONS AND PRECAUTIONS

Contraindicated in: ■ Hypersensitivity ■ Self-diagnosed depression ■ Bipolar disorder.

Use Cautiously in: ■ Pregnancy, lactation, or children (safety not established).

ADVERSE REACTIONS AND SIDE EFFECTS

CNS: agitation, manic reactions (in patients with bipolar disorder).
GI: GI distress.

INTERACTIONS

Drug-Drug: ■ Should not be used concurrently with MAO inhibitors.

ROUTE AND DOSAGE

■ **PO (Adults):** *Depression*—200 mg once or twice daily, adjusted upward over 2 wk (range 200–1600 mg/day); *liver disorders*—1600 mg/day; *osteoarthritis*— 400–1600 mg/day.

AVAILABILITY

TIME/ACTION PROFILE (antidepressant action)

	ONSET	PEAK	DURATION
PO	unknown	unknown	unknown

NURSING IMPLICATIONS

ASSESSMENT

- Assess mental status for symptoms of depression prior to and periodically during therapy; should not be used for self-diagnosed depression.
- Assess symptoms of pain and fatigue prior to and periodically during therapy.

POTENTIAL NURSING DIAGNOSES

■ Ineffective individual coping (Indications).
■ Knowledge deficit related to medication regimen.

IMPLEMENTATION

■ **General Info:** Only enteric-coated formulations are recommended due to bioavailability problems.
■ **PO:** Initial dose should be 200 mg once or twice daily to minimize GI disturbances. Dosage may be adjusted upward over 1–2 wks depending on response and tolerance.

PATIENT/FAMILY TEACHING

❑ Instruct patient to take SAMe according to directions.

EVALUATION

■ Decrease in symptoms of depression.

TENECTEPLASE
(te-**nek**-te-plase)
TNKase

CLASSIFICATION(S):
Thrombolytic agents (plasminogen activator)

Pregnancy Category C

INDICATIONS

■ Reduction of mortality associated with acute myocardial infarctions (AMI).

ACTION

■ Converts plasminogen to plasmin, which is then able to degrade fibrin present in clots. Directly activates plasminogen. Therapeutic Effects: ■ Lysis of thrombi in coronary arteries, with preservation of myocardium and decreased mortality.

PHARMACOKINETICS

Absorption: IV administration results in complete bioavailability.

Distribution: Unknown.

Metabolism and Excretion: Mostly metabolized by the liver.

Half-life: *Initial phase* —20–24 min; *terminal phase* — 90–130 min.

CONTRAINDICATIONS AND PRECAUTIONS

Contraindicated in: ■ Active internal bleeding ■ History of cerebrovascular accident, recent CNS trauma or surgery, neoplasm, or arteriovenous malformation (within 2 months) ■ Severe uncontrolled hypertension ■ Known bleeding tendencies ■ Hypersensitivity.

Use Cautiously in: ■ Recent major surgery, trauma, GI, or GU bleeding ■ Cerebrovacular disease ■ Hypertension (BP ≥180 mm Hg and or diastolic ≥110 mm Hg) ■ Presence or high likelihood of left heart thrombus ■ Subacute bacterial endocarditis or acute pericarditis ■ Hemostatic defect especially when associated with severe hepatic or renal disease ■ Severe hepatic dysfunction ■ Geriatric patients (increased risk of intracranial bleeding) ■ Hemorrhagic ophthalmic conditions ■ Septic phlebitis or occluded AV cannula at infected site ■ Concurrent warfarin therapy or recent therapy with glycoptrotein (GP) IIb/IIIa inhibitors (abciximab, eptifibatide, tirofiban) ■ Pregnancy, lactation, or children (safety not established).

ADVERSE REACTIONS AND SIDE EFFECTS

Adverse reactions are frequently sequelae of underlying disease.

CV: ARRHYTHMIAS , CARDIOGENIC SHOCK , CARDIAC TAMPONADE ,EMBOLISM ,HEART FAILURE ,MYOCARDIAL INFARCTION, MYOCARDIAL RUPTURE, PERICARDITIS , PERICARDIAL EFFUSION , PULMONARY EDEMA ,RECURRENT MYOCARDIAL ISCHEMIA ,THROMBOSIS , hypotension.

GI: nausea, vomiting.

Hemat: BLEEDING .

Misc: allergic reactions including ANAPHYLAXIS, fever.

INTERACTIONS

Drug-Drug: ■ **Aspirin**, **NSAIDs**, **warfarin**, **heparin** and **heparin-like agents**, **abciximab**, **eptifibatide**, **tirofiban**, **clopidogrel**, **ticlopidine**, or **dipyridamole**—concurrent use may increase the risk of bleeding, although these agents are frequently used together or in sequence ■ Risk of bleeding may be increased by concurrent use of **cefamandole**, **cefotetan**, **cefoperazone**, **plicamycin**, or **valproic acid**.

ROUTE AND DOSAGE

■ **IV (Adults <60 kg):** 30 mg
■ **IV (Adults ≥60 kg and <70 kg):** 35 mg
■ **IV (Adults ≥70 kg and <80 kg):** 40 mg
■ **IV (Adults ≥80 kg and <90 kg):** 45 mg
■ **IV (Adults ≥90 kg):** 50 mg

AVAILABILITY

■ *Powder for injection:* 50 mg/vial with 10 ml syringe and TwinPak Dual Cannula Device, and 10 ml vial of sterile water for injection.

TIME/ACTION PROFILE (fibrinolysis)

	ONSET	PEAK	DURATION
IV	rapid	unknown	unknown

NURSING IMPLICATIONS

ASSESSMENT

■ **General Info:** Begin therapy as soon as possible after the onset of symptoms.

❑ Assess patients for bleeding every 15 min during the 1st hr, every 15–30 min during the next 8 hr, and at least every 4 hr for the duration of therapy. Frank bleeding may occur from invasive sites or body orifices. Internal bleeding may also occur (decreased neurologic status, abdominal pain with coffee-ground emesis or black tarry stools, joint pain). If uncontrolled bleeding occurs, stop tenecteplase immediately.

❑ Monitor vital signs, including temperature, every 4 hr during course of therapy. Do not use lower extremities to measure blood pressure. Notify physician if systolic BP >180 mmHg or diastolic BP >110 mmHg. Tenecteplase should not be given if hypertension is uncontrolled. Inform physician if hypotension occurs. Hypotension may result from the drug, hemorrhage, or cardiogenic shock.

❑ Assess neurologic status throughout therapy. Altered sensorium or mental changes may be indicative of intracranial bleeding.

■ **Coronary Thrombosis:** Monitor ECG continuously in patients with coronary thrombosis for significant arrhythmias. Antiarrhythmics may be ordered prior to or during alteplase therapy to prevent reperfusion arrhythmias. Cardiac enzymes should be monitored. Coronary angiography or radionuclide myocardial scanning may be used to assess effectiveness of therapy.

❑ Assess intensity, character, location, and radiation of chest pain. Note presence of associated symptoms (nausea, vomiting, diaphoresis). Administer analgesics as ordered by physician. Notify physician if chest pain is unrelieved or recurs.

❑ Monitor heart and breath sounds frequently. Inform physician of signs of congestive heart failure (rales/crackles, dyspnea, S heart sound, jugular venous distention, elevated CVP).

■ *Lab Test Considerations:* Monitor hematocrit, hemoglobin, platelet count, prothrombin time, thrombin time, activated partial thromboplastin time, and fibrinolytic activity prior to and frequently throughout therapy. Bleeding time may be assessed prior to therapy if patient has received platelet aggregation inhibitors.

❑ Obtain type and crossmatch of blood and have blood available at all times in case of hemorrhage.

❑ Stools should be tested for occult blood loss and urine tested for hematuria periodically during therapy.

■ *Toxicity and Overdose:* If local bleeding occurs, apply pressure to site. If severe internal bleeding occurs, discontinue infusion. Clotting factors and/or blood volume may be restored through infusions of whole blood, packed RBCs, fresh frozen plasma, or cryoprecipitate. Do not administer dextran, as it has antiplatelet activity. Aminocaproic acid (Amicar) may be used as an antidote.

POTENTIAL NURSING DIAGNOSES

■ Pain, acute.
■ Altered tissue perfusion (Indications).
■ Injury, risk for, high risk for (Adverse Reactions).

IMPLEMENTATION

■ **General Info:** Tenecteplase should be used only in settings where hematologic function and clinical response can be adequately monitored. Avoid IM injections and unnecessary venipunctures. Apply pressure to all arterial and venous punctures for at least 30 min. Avoid venipunctures at noncompressible sites (e.g., jugular and subclavian sites).

❑ Avoid invasive procedures, such as IM injections or arterial punctures, with this therapy. If such procedures must be performed, apply pressure to all arterial and venous puncture sites for at least 30 min. Avoid venipunctures at noncompressible sites (jugular vein, subclavian site).

❑ Systemic anticoagulation with heparin is usually begun several hours after the completion of thrombolytic therapy.

❑ Acetaminophen may be ordered to control fever.

■ **IV:** Prior to therapy start two IV lines: one for tenecteplase, the other for any additional IV infusions.

■ **Intermittent Infusion:** Vials are packaged with sterile water for injection (without preservatives) to be used as diluent. Do not use bacteriostatic water for injection. Do not discard shield assembly. To reconstitute aseptically withdraw 10 ml of diluent and inject into the tenectplase vial, directing the stream into the powder. Slight foaming may occur; large bubbles will dissipate if left standing undisturbed for several minutes. Swirl gently until contents are completely dissolved; do not shake. Solution containing 5 mg/ml is clear and colorless to pale yellow. Withdraw dose from reconstituted vial with the syringe and discard unused portion. Once dose is in syringe, stand the shield vertically on a flat surface (with green side down) and passively recap the red hub cannula. Remove the entire shield assembly, including the red hub cannula, by twisting counter clockwise. Shield assembly also contains the clear-ended blunt plastic cannula; retain for split septum IV access. Reconstitute immediately before use. May be refrigerated and administered within 8 hrs.

■ *Rate:* Administer as a single IV bolus over 5 seconds.

■ **Y-Site Incompatibility:** Precipate forms in line when administered with dextrose-containing solutions. Flush line with saline-containing solution prior to and following administration of tenecteplase.

■ **Additive Incompatibility:** Do not admix.

PATIENT/FAMILY TEACHING

❑ Explain to patient and family the purpose of tenecteplase and the need for close monitoring.

❑ Advise patient to remain on bed rest and to avoid unnecessary procedures such as shaving and vigorous toothbrushing for 24 hr.

❑ Instruct patient to report signs of hypersensitivity and bleeding promptly.

EVALUATION

Effectiveness of therapy can be demonstrated by: ■ Restoration of coronary perfusion resulting in limitation of infarct size and decrease in complications, such as CHF.

TINZAPARIN
(tin-**za**-par-in)
Innohep

CLASSIFICATION(S):
Anticoagulants (antithrombotic)

Pregnancy Category B

INDICATIONS

■ Treatment of acute symptomatic deep vein thrombosis (DVT) with or without pulmonary embolism; given in conjunction with warfarin.

ACTION

■ Potentiates the inhibitory effect of antithrombin on factor X and thrombin ■ Tinzaparin is a low molecular weight heparin. Therapeutic Effects: ■ Prevention of thrombus formation.

PHARMACOKINETICS

Absorption: Well absorbed following SC administration.

Distribution: Unknown.

Metabolism and Excretion: Partially metabolized; elimination is primarily renal.

Half-life: 3.9 hr.

CONTRAINDICATIONS AND PRECAUTIONS

Contraindicated in: ■ Hypersensitivity; including hypersensitivity to bisulfites (contains metabisulfite), benzyl alcohol, or pork products ■ Active major bleeding ■ History of heparin-induced thrombocytopenia.

Use Cautiously in: ■ Geriatric patients (may have increased sensitivity) ■ Renal insufficiency ■ Diabetic retinopathy ■ Concurrent use of platelet inhibitors, oral anticoagulants, or thrombolytics (increased risk of bleeding) ■ Pregnancy (benzyl alcohol in formulation may cause gasping syndrome in neonate; use during pregnancy only if clearly needed) ■ Lactation or children (safety not established).

Exercise Extreme Caution in: ■ Epidural or spinal anesthesia or spinal puncture especially when used concurrently with indwelling epidural catheters, traumatic or repeated epidural or spinal puncture, or concurrent use of drugs that may increase the risk of bleeding (other anticoagulants, antiplatelet agents, or NSAIDs); increases the risk of spinal/epidural hematomas and paralysis ■ Bacterial endocarditis ■ Severe uncontrolled hypertension ■ Congenital/acquired bleeding disorders including hepatic failure and amyloidosis ■ Active ulcerative/agiodysplastic GI disease ■ Shortly after brain/spinal/ophthalmologic surgery ■ Hemorrhagic stroke.

ADVERSE REACTIONS AND SIDE EFFECTS

GI: increased liver function tests.

Hemat: BLEEDING, thrombocytopenia.

Local: ecchymoses, hematoma, local irritation, pain.

Misc: hypersensitivity reactions.

INTERACTIONS

Drug-Drug: ■ Concurrent use of **platelet inhibitors**, **warfarin**, or **thrombolytics** (increased risk of bleeding).

ROUTE AND DOSAGE

■ **SC (Adults):** 175 anti-Xa IU/kg once daily for at least 6 days and until adequate anticoagulation is achieved with warfarin.

AVAILABILITY

■ *Solution for injection:* 20,000 anti-Xa units/ml in 2-ml vials ■ Cost: To come.

TIME/ACTION PROFILE

	ONSET	PEAK	DURATION
SC	rapid		24 hr

NURSING IMPLICATIONS

ASSESSMENT

❏ Assess patient for signs of bleeding and hemorrhage (bleeding gums; nose bleed; unusual bruising; black, tarry stool; hematuria; fall in hematocrit or blood pressure; guaiac-positive stools). Notify physician if these occur.

❏ Observe injection sites for hematoma, ecchymosis, or inflammation.

❏ Monitor neurologic status frequently for signs of neurologic impairment. May require urgent treatment.

■ *Lab Test Considerations:* Monitor CBC, platelet count, and stools for occult blood periodically throughout therapy. If thrombocytopenia occurs, monitor closely. If platelet count is <100,000/mm³, discontinue tinzaparin. If hematocrit decreases unexpectedly, assess patient for potential bleeding sites.

❏ Special monitoring of clotting times (PT and PTT) is not necessary. Patients receiving both tinzaparin and warfarin should have blood for PT/international normalized ratio (INR) drawn just prior to the next scheduled dose of tinzaparin.

❏ May cause asymptomatic increases in transaminase levels (AST, ALT).

POTENTIAL NURSING DIAGNOSES

■ Altered tissue perfusion (Indications).

■ Injury, risk for (Side Effects).

■ Knowledge deficit, related to medication regimen (Patient/Family Teaching).

IMPLEMENTATION

■ **General Info:** Tinzaparin cannot be used interchangeably (unit for unit) with unfractionated heparin or other low–molecular weight heparins.

❏ Tinzaparin should be administered daily for at least 6 days and until patient is adequately anticoagulated with warfarin (INR at least 2.0 for 2 consecutive days). Warfarin therapy should be started within 1–3 days of tinzaparin initiation.

❏ Solution is clear and colorless to slightly yellow; do not administer solutions that are discolored or contain particulate matter.

❏ Multiple dose vial contains benzyl alcohol; use with caution in pregnant women.

■ **SC:** Administer deep SC while patient is sitting or lying down. Tinzaparin injection should be alternated between the left and right anterolateral and posterolateral abdominal wall. Rotate injection sites daily.   Inject entire length of needle at a 45° or 90° angle while lifting and holding skin between thumb and forefinger; hold the skin throughout the injection. To minimize bruising, do not rub injection site following the injection.

❑ Do not administer IM or IV.

■ **Syringe Incompatibility:** Do not mix with other injections or infusions.

PATIENT/FAMILY TEACHING

❑ Advise patient to report any symptoms of unusual bleeding or bruising, dizziness, itching, rash, fever, swelling, or difficulty breathing to health care professional immediately.

❑ Instruct patient not to take aspirin or other NSAIDs without consulting health care professional while on tinzaparin therapy.

EVALUATION

Effectiveness of therapy can be demonstrated by: ■ Improvement in symptoms of acute deep vein thrombosis.

Additional Drugs

Generic name Trade name(s) Classification Pregnancy category Scheduled substance	Indications	Adverse Reactions and Side Effects*	Route and Dosage
albumin Albuminar, Albutein, Buminate, normal human serum albumin, Plasbumin *Volume expanders* Pregnancy category C	Expansion of plasma volume/maintenance of cardiac output in situations associated with fluid volume deficit, including shock, hemorrhage, and burns. Temporary replacement of albumin in diseases associated with low levels of plasma proteins, such as nephrotic syndrome or end-stage liver disease.	**CNS:** headache. **CV:** PULMONARY EDEMA, fluid overload, hypertension, hypotension, tachycardia. **GI:** increased salivation, nausea, vomiting. **Derm:** rash, urticaria. **MS:** back pain. **Misc:** chills, fever, flushing.	***Shock (5% Albumin)*** IV **(Adults):** 500 ml, may be repeated within 30 min. IV **(Children):** 50 ml. IV **(Infants and Neonates):** 10–20 ml/kg as a 5% solution. ***Hypoproteinemia (25% Albumin)*** IV **(Adults):** 50–75 g. IV **(Children):** 25 g. ***Acute Nephrosis (25% Albumin)*** IV **(Adults):** 100 ml daily with loop diuretic for 7–10 days (until response to corticosteroids).
NOTES: **Contraindications:** Allergic reactions to albumin; severe anemia; congestive heart failure; normal or increased intravascular volume. **Cautions:** Severe hepatic or renal disease; dehydration.			
alfentanil Ridaura *Opioid analgesics (agonists)* Schedule II Pregnancy category C	Analgesic adjunct when given in increasing doses in the maintenance of anesthesia with barbiturate/nitrous oxide/oxygen. Analgesic when administered by continuous IV infusion with nitrous oxide/oxygen while maintaining general anesthesia. Primary induction of anesthesia when endotracheal intubation and mechanical ventilation are required.	**CNS:** dizziness, sleepiness. **EENT:** blurred vision. **Resp:** apnea, respiratory depression. **CV:** bradycardia, hypertension, hypotension, tachycardia, arrhythmias. **GI:** nausea, vomiting. **MS:** thoracic muscle rigidity, skeletal muscle rigidity.	***Incremental Injection (Duration of Anesthesia <30 min)—Induction Period*** IV **(Adults):** 8–20 mcg/kg. ***Incremental Injection (Duration of Anesthesia <30 min)—Maintenance Period*** IV **(Adults):** 3–5 mcg/kg increments or 0.5–1 mcg/kg/min (total dose 8–40 mcg/kg). ***Incremental Injection (Duration of Anesthesia 30–60 min)—Induction Period*** IV **(Adults):** 20–50 mcg/kg. ***Incremental Injection (Duration of Anesthesia 30–60 min)—Maintenance Period*** IV **(Adults):** 5–15 mcg/kg increments (up to total dose of 75 mg/kg).

{ } available in Canada only. *CAPITALS indicate life-threatening, underlines indicate most frequent

(continued)

ADDITIONAL DRUGS (CONTINUED)

Generic name Trade name(s) Classification Pregnancy category Scheduled substance	Indications	Adverse Reactions and Side Effects*	Route and Dosage
alfentanil (continued) Ridaura *Opioid analgesics (agonists)* Schedule II Pregnancy category C			***Continuous Infusion (Duration of Anesthesia >45 min) –Induction Period*** IV (Adults): 50–75 mcg/kg. ***Continuous Infusion (Duration of Anesthesia >45 min)–Maintenance Period*** IV (Adults): 0.5–3.0 mcg/kg/min (average infusion rate 1–1.5 mcg/kg/min). Infusion rate should be decreased by 30–50% after first hour of maintenance. If lightening occurs, infusion rate may be increased up to 4 mcg/kg/min or boluses of 7 mcg/kg may be administered. ***Anesthetic Induction (Duration of Anesthesia >45 min)*** IV (Adults): 130–245 mcg/kg followed by 0.5–1.5 mcg/kg/min or general anesthesia. ***Monitored Anesthesia Care (MAC)–Induction Period*** IV (Adults): 3–8 mcg/kg. ***Monitored Anesthesia Care (MAC)–Maintenance Period*** IV (Adults): 3–5 mcg/kg q 5–20 min or followed by 0.25–1 mcg/kg/min (total dose 3–40 mg/kg).
amobarbital Amytal *Anticonvulsants Anti-anxiety and sedative/ hypnotic agents* Schedule II Pregnancy category D	Preoperative sedative and in other situations in which sedation may be required. Hypnotic	**CNS:** drowsiness, hangover, delirium, depression, excitation, lethargy, syncope, vertigo. **Resp:** BRONCHOSPASM (IV only), LARYNGOSPASM (IV only), respiratory depression. **CV:** bradycardia, hypotension. **GI:** constipation, diarrhea, nausea, vomiting.	PO (Adults): *Sedative* 50–300 mg/day in divided doses; *hypnotic*—65–200 mg at bedtime; *preoperative sedation*—200 mg 1–2 hr before surgery. PO (Children): *Daytime sedation*—2 mg/kg or 60 mg/m² 3 times daily; *preoperative sedation*—2–6 mg/kg, up to 100 mg/dose.

NOTES: Contraindications: Hypersensitivity or known intolerance. **Cautions:** Geriatric patients, debilitated or severely ill patients, diabetic patients, severe pulmonary or hepatic disease, CNS tumors, increased intracranial pressure, head trauma, adrenal insufficiency, undiagnosed abdominal pain, hypothyroidism, alcoholism, cardiac disease (arrhythmias); pregnancy, lactation, and children <12yr (safety not established).

		IV (Adults): *Sedative*—30–50 mg 2–3 times daily; *hypnotic*—65–200 mg.
		IV (Children 6 yr): 65–500 mg (3–5 mg/kg), depending on response.
	Derm: exfoliative dermatitis, photosensitivity, rashes, urticaria.	IM (Children <6 yr): 3–5 mg/kg (125 mg/m²)/dose.
	Local: pain or sterile abscess at IM site, phlebitis at IV site.	IM (Children 6 yr): *Hypnotic*—2–3 mg/kg/dose.
	MS: arthralgia, myalgia.	IM (Children <6 yr): *Hypnotic*—2–3 mg/kg; *anticonvulsant*—3–5 mg/kg (125 mg/m²)/dose.
	Misc: hypersensitivity reactions including STEVENS-JOHNSON SYNDROME.	

NOTES: Contraindications: Hypersensitivity; comatose patients; severe uncontrolled pain, pregnancy and lactation; pre-existing CNS depression, pre-existing respiratory depression; patients with hepatic or renal impairment. **Interactions:** ↑ CNS depression with other CNS. MAO inhibitors ↑ sedation. May ↓ the effectiveness of oral contraceptives, chloramphenicol, acebutolol, propranolol, metoprolol, timolol, doxycycline, corticosteroids, tricyclic antidepressants, phenothiazines, theophylline, and quinidine.

amoxapine Asendin *Antidepressants (tricyclic)*	Treatment of depression accompanied by anxiety, often used in conjunction with psychotherapy	CNS: NEUROLEPTIC MALIGNANT SYNDROME, fatigue, sedation, extrapyramidal reactions, tardive dyskinesia. EENT: blurred vision, dry eyes, dry mouth. CV: ARRHYTHMIAS, hypotension, ECG changes. GI: constipation, increased appetite, paralytic ileus. GU: testicular swelling, urinary retention. Derm: photosensitivity, rash. Endo: gynecomastia, sexual dysfunction. Hemat: blood dyscrasias. Misc: fever, weight gain.	PO (Adults): 50 mg 2–3 times daily, increase to 100 mg 2–3 times daily by end of 1 week (not to exceed 300 mg daily in outpatients, 600 mg daily in divided doses in hospitalized patients). Once optimal dose is achieved, may be given as a single bedtime dose; one single dose to exceed 300 mg. PO (Geriatric Patients): 25 mg 2–3 times daily, may be increased to 50 mg 2–3 times daily (not >300 mg/day).

NOTES: Contraindications: Glaucoma; pregnancy and lactation. **Cautions:** Geriatric patients; cardiovascular disease; prostatic hypertrophy; history of seizures; children <16 yr. **Interactions:** May cause fatal reactions when used with MAO inhibitors (avoid concurrent use; discontinue 2 wk before amoxapine). May ↑ the effects of other antidepressants, phenothiazines, carbamazepine, and type IC antiarrhythmics. Effects may be ↑ by cimetidine, quinidine, amiodarone, ritonavir, oral contraceptives, or phenothiazines. Concurrent use with SSRI antidepressants may cause toxicity; fluoxetine should be stopped 5 wk before amoxapin. May prevent response to guanethidine. Clonidine may cause hypertensive crisis and ↑ risk of extrapyramidal reactions. Concurrent use with levodopa may result in ↓ absorption of levodopa or hypertension Effects may be ↓ by rifapentine, rifampin, rifabutin. ↑ risk of extrapyramidal reactions with other drugs causing extrapyramidal reactions.

anileridine [Leritine] *Opioid analgesics (agonists)* Pregnancy category UK	Moderate to severe pain. Relief of apprehension in congestive heart failure (CHF). Anesthesia adjunct. Analgesic during labor. Preoperative sedation.	CNS: dizziness, euphoria, excitement, nervousness, restlessness. EENT: disturbed vision. Resp: RESPIRATORY DEPRESSION. GI: constipation, dry mouth, nausea, vomiting. Derm: flushing, itching, sweating. Misc: physical dependence, psychological dependence, tolerance.	*Analgesia/Preoperative Use/Supplement to Anesthesia* PO (Adults): 25–50 mg q 6 hr; if pain is extremely severe, initial dose may be 50 mg or more frequent intervals may be used but should be reserved for nonambulatory patients. SC, IM (Adults): *Analgesia*—25–50 mg q 4–6 hr; for more severe pain, 75–100 mg and smaller, more frequent doses used (not to exceed 200 mg/24 hr). *Preoperative use*—50–75 mg.

{ } available in Canada only. *CAPITALS indicate life-threatening; underlines indicate most frequent

(continued)

ADDITIONAL DRUGS (CONTINUED)

Generic name Trade name(s) *Classification* Pregnancy category Scheduled substance	Indications	Adverse Reactions and Side Effects*	Route and Dosage
aniteridine (continued) [Leritine] *Opioid analgesics (agonists)* Pregnancy category UK			**IV (Adults):** *Supplement to anesthesia*—5–10 mg followed by 0.6 mg/min. *Analgesia During Labor* **IV, IM, SC (Adults):** 50 mg IM or SC; may be repeated in 3–4 hr (not to exceed 100–200 mg total dose) or 40 mg IM or SC given concurrently with 10 mg IV.

NOTES: Contraindications: Hypersensitivity; some products contain bisulfites and should be avoided in patients with known intolerance. **Cautions :** Head trauma, increased intracranial pressure; severe renal, hepatic, or pulmonary disease; hypothyroidism; adrenal insufficiency; alcoholism; geriatric/ debilitated patients; undiagnosed abdominal pain; prostatic hypertrophy; pregnancy or lactation; children <12 yr (safety not established). **Interactions:** Use with extreme caution in patients receiving MAO inhibitors (may cause severe reactions; ↓ initial dose to 25% of usual dose). ↑ CNS depression with other CNS depressants. Partial-antagonist opioids may cause opioid withdrawal in physically dependent patients. Buprenorphine, dezocine, nalbuphine, and pentazocine may ↓ analgesia.

antihemophilic factor Alphanate, Bioclate, Helixate, Humate-P, HYATE:C, Koate-HP, Kogenate, Monoclate-P Profilate HP, Recombinate, ReFacto *Hemostatic agents* Pregnancy category C	Management of hemophilia A associated with a deficiency of factor VIII. Antihemophilic factor, AHF (porcine, HYATE:C), is used in patients with antibodies to factor VIII. Some products (Humate-P) are used in the management of von Willebrand's disease that has not responded adequately to desmopressin.	**CNS:** headache, lethargy, loss of consciousness. **EENT:** visual disturbances. **CV:** chest tightness, hypotension, tachycardia. **GI:** nausea, vomiting. **Derm:** flushing, urticaria. **Hemat:** intravascular hemolysis. **MS:** back pain. **Neuro:** paresthesia. **Misc:** allergic reactions, hepatitis B, C, D, or HIV virus infection (small risk), jaundice, rigor.	Consult individual product information for more specific dosing information. Dosage may be calculated using the following formula: Dose AHF (units) = body weight (kg) × desired AHF increase (% normal) × 0.5. Each unit of AHF/kg may be expected to produce a 2% rise in factor VIII activity.

NOTES: Contraindications: Hypersensitivity to hamster, murine, or bovine proteins (in recombinant and monoclonal antibody products); hypersensitivity to porcine products (HYATE:C only).
Cautions: Hypersensitivity to AHF; pregnancy (safety not established).

atovaquone Mepron *Anti-infective agents (antiprotozoal)* Pregnancy category C	Treatment of mild to moderate *Pneumocystis carinii* pneumonia (PCP) in patients who are unable to tolerate trimethoprim/sulfamethoxazole. Prophylaxis of PCP	**CNS:** headache, insomnia. **Resp:** cough. **GI:** diarrhea, nausea, vomiting. **Derm:** rash. **Misc:** fever.	**Treatment** **PO (Adults):** 750 mg twice daily for 21 days. **Prevention** **PO (Adults and Adolescents 13–16 yr):** 1500 mg once daily.

NOTES: Contraindications: Hypersensitivity. **Cautions:** Decreased hepatic/renal/cardiac function; GI disorders; pregnancy; lactation; or children.

auranofin
Ridaura
Antirheumatic agents (disease-modifying)
Pregnancy category C

Treatment of progressive rheumatoid arthritis resistant to conventional therapy.

CNS: dizziness, headache, syncope.
EENT: corneal gold deposits, corneal ulcerations.
Resp: pneumonitis.
CV: bradycardia.
GI: abdominal pain, cramping, diarrhea, metallic taste, stomatitis, anorexia, dysphagia, hepatitis, dyspepsia, flatulence, nausea, vomiting.
Derm: dermatitis, rash, photosensitivity, pruritus.
Hemat: AGRANULOCYTOSIS, APLASTIC ANEMIA, thrombocytopenia, eosinophilia, leukopenia.
Misc: allergic reactions, including ANAPHYLAXIS, ANGIONEUROTIC EDEMA, nitritoid reactions.

PO (Adults): 6 mg/day in 1–2 doses; may increase to 9 mg/day in 3 divided doses if no improvement after 6 mo.

NOTES: Contraindications: Hypersensitivity; severe hepatic/renal dysfunction; previous heavy metal toxicity; history of colitis or exfoliative dermatitis; tuberculosis; CHF; systemic lupus erythematosus; recent radiation therapy; pregnancy or lactation. **Cautions:** History of blood dyscrasias; hypertension ; rashes.

aurothioglucose
Solganol
Antirheumatic agents (disease-modifying)
Pregnancy category C

Treatment of progressive rheumatoid arthritis resistant to conventional therapy

CNS: dizziness, headache, syncope.
EENT: corneal gold deposits, corneal ulcerations.
Resp: pneumonitis.
CV: bradycardia.
GI: abdominal pain, cramping, diarrhea, metallic taste, stomatitis, anorexia, dysphagia, hepatitis, dyspepsia, flatulence, nausea, vomiting.
Derm: dermatitis, rash, photosensitivity, pruritus.
Hemat: AGRANULOCYTOSIS, APLASTIC ANEMIA, thrombocytopenia, eosinophilia, leukopenia.
Neuro: neuropathy
Misc: allergic reactions, including ANAPHYLAXIS, ANGIONEUROTIC EDEMA, nitritoid reactions

IM (Adults): 10 mg 1st wk, then 25 mg 2nd and 3rd wks, then 25–50 mg/wk until improvement or toxicity occurs (up to 1 g total). Maintenance dose is 25–50 mg q 2 wk for up to 20 wk, then q 3–4 wk.
IM (Children 6–12 yr): 2.5 mg 1st week, then 6.25 mg 2nd and 3rd wks, then 12.5 mg weekly until a total of 200–250 mg has been given. Maintenance dose is 6.25–12.5 mg q 3–4 wk.
IM (Children): 10 mg initially, followed 1 wk later by 1 mg/kg q 2 wk for up to 20 wk, then q 3–4 wk

NOTES: Contraindications: Hypersensitivity; severe hepatic/renal dysfunction; previous heavy metal toxicity; history of colitis or exfoliative dermatitis; tuberculosis; CHF; systemic lupus erythematosus; recent radiation therapy; pregnancy or lactation. **Cautions:** History of blood dyscrasias; hypertension , rashes.

aztreonam
Azactam
Anti-infective (monobactam)
Pregnancy category B

Treatment of serious gram-negative infections including: bone and joint infections, septicemia, skin and skin structure infections, intra-abdominal infections, gynecologic infections, respiratory tract infections, urinary tract infections.

CNS: SEIZURES.
GI: altered taste (IV only), diarrhea, nausea, vomiting.
Derm: rashes.
Local: pain at IM site, phlebitis at IV site.
Misc: allergic reactions including ANAPHYLAXIS, superinfection.

IM, IV (Adults): *Most infections*—0.5–2 g q 6–12 hr; *life-threatening infections*—2 g q 6–8 hr; *urinary tract infections* 0.5–1 g q 8–12 hr.
IM, IV (Children 9 mo–16 yr): *Most infections*—30 mg/kg q 6–8 hr; *serious infections*—50 mg/kg q 4–6 hr.

(continued)

() available in Canada only. *CAPITALS indicate life-threatening, underlines indicate most frequent

ADDITIONAL DRUGS (CONTINUED)

Generic name Trade name(s) *Classification* Pregnancy category Scheduled substance	Indications	Adverse Reactions and Side Effects*	Route and Dosage
aztreonam (continued) Azactam *Anti-infective (monobactam)* Pregnancy category B	Useful for treatment of multiresistant strains of some bacteria including anaerobic gram-negative pathogens.		
NOTES: Contraindications: Hypersensitivity. Cross-sensitivity with penicillins or cephalosporins may occur rarely. **Cautions:** Renal impairment; pregnancy, lactation, and children.			
bitolterol Tornalate *Bronchodilators (adrenergic agonist)* Pregnancy category C	Used as a quick-relief agent in the management of reversible airway disease caused by asthma or COPD.	**CNS:** nervousness, restlessness, tremor, headache, insomnia, light-headedness. **Resp:** PARADOXICAL BRONCHOSPASM. **CV:** chest pain, palpitations, tachycardia, arrhythmias, hypertension. **GI:** nausea, vomiting. **Endo:** hyperglycemia, hypokalemia. **Neuro:** tremor.	*Metered-Dose Inhaler* Inhaln (**Adults and Children ≥12 yr**): *Treatment*—2 inhalations (1–3 min apart), followed by an additional inhalation if needed (not to exceed 2 inhalations q 4 hr or 3 inhalations q 6 hr). *Prophylaxis* — inhalations q 8 hr (370 mcg/spray). *Solution for Inhalation* Inhaln (**Adults and Children ≥12 yr**): One treatment 3 times daily; interval between treatments should not 4 hr (not to exceed 8 mg/day by intermittent flow nebulization or 16 mg/day by continuous flow nebulization).
NOTES: Contraindications: Hypersensitivity to adrenergic amines; known alcohol intolerance. **Cautions:** Cardiovascular disease; hyperthyroidism; diabetes; glaucoma; geriatric patients; pregnancy, lactation, and children <2 yr. Excessive use may cause tolerance and paradoxical bronchospasm.			
bretylium [Bretylol], Breylol *Antiarrhythmic agent (group III)* Pregnancy category C	Treatment of ventricular tachycardia. Prophylaxis against ventricular fibrillation. Treatment of other serious ventricular arrhythmias resistant to lidocaine.	**CNS:** dizziness, faintness. **EENT:** nasal stuffiness. **CV:** postural hypotension, angina, bradycardia, transient hypertension. **GI:** nausea, vomiting, diarrhea.	*Ventricular Fibrillation/Ventricular Tachycardia* IV (**Adults**): 5 mg/kg bolus over 15–30 sec initially; if no response, increase to 10 mg/kg, repeat as necessary (not to exceed 30 mg/kg/24 hr). Maintenance: 5–10 mg/kg q 6 hr or 1–2 mg/min continuous infusion. *Other Ventricular Arrhythmias* IV (**Adults**): 5–10 mg/kg q 1–2 hr; then q 6 hr as maintenance; may also be given as a continuous infusion at 1–2 mg/min. IM (**Adults**): 5–10 mg/kg, repeat q 1-2 hr if arrhythmia persists, then q 6-8 hr.
NOTES: Cautions: Geriatric patients; suspected digoxin toxicity; fixed cardiac; renal insufficiency; pregnancy, lactation, and children.			

calfactant Infasurf *Pulmonary surfactant* Pregnancy category UK	Treatment and prophylaxis of respiratory distress syndrome (RDS, hyaline membrane disease) in premature infants.	**Intratracheal (Infants):** *Prophylaxis*—3 ml/kg as soon as possible after birth given as 2 doses of 1.5 ml/kg. *Treatment*—3 ml/kg birthweight given as 2 doses of 1.5 ml/kg up to a total of 3 doses 12 hours apart.

Resp: Airway obstruction bradycardia, cyanosis, reflux of surfactant into endotracheal tube, require-ment for mechanical ventilation/reintubation.

NOTES: Contraindications/Cautions: None significant.

casanthranol *Laxatives (stimulants)* Pregnancy category UK	Treatment of constipation. Particularly useful when constipation is secondary to prolonged bedrest or constipating drugs. Casanthranol is available only in combination with other laxatives.	**PO (Adults):** 30–90 mg once daily. **PO (Children 2–11 yr):** 15–45 mg once daily. **PO (Children <2 yr):** 7.5–22.5 mg once daily.

GI: abdominal cramps, nausea, diarrhea.
GU: discoloration of urine.
F and E: hypokalemia (with chronic use).

NOTES: **Contraindications:** Hypersensitivity; abdominal pain/obstruction/nausea/vomiting; pregnancy or lactation. **Cautions:** Severe cardiovascular disease; anal/rectal fissures. Excessive or prolonged use may lead to dependence.

cascara sagrada *Laxatives (stimulants)* Pregnancy category UK	Treatment of constipation. Particularly useful when constipation is secondary to prolonged bedrest or constipating drugs. Casanthranol is available only in combination with other laxatives.	**PO (Adults):** 300 mg–1 g once daily. **PO (Children 2–11 yr):** 150–500 mg once daily. **PO (Children <2 yr):** 75–250 mg once daily.

GI: abdominal cramps, nausea, diarrhea.
GU: discoloration of urine.
F and E: hypokalemia (with chronic use).

NOTES: **Contraindications:** Hypersensitivity, abdominal pain, obstruction, nausea, or vomiting; pregnancy or lactation. **Cautions:** Severe cardiovascular disease; anal or rectal fissures. Excessive or prolonged use may lead to dependence.

chloramphenicol Chloromycetin, (Novochlorocap) *Anti-infective agents (miscellaneous)* Pregnancy category UK	Management of the following serious infections when less toxic agents cannot be used: skin and soft-tissue infections, intraabdominal infections, CNS infections (including meningitis), and bacteremia	**PO, IV (Adults):** 12.5 mg/kg q 6 hr (up to 4 g/day). **PO, IV (Infants >2 wk and Children):** *Most infections*—12 mg/kg q 6 hr *or* 25 mg/kg q 12 hr. *Bacteremia/meningitis*—up to 75–100 mg/kg/day. **PO, IV (Infants Premature and Full Term, 2 wk):** *Most infections*—6.25 mg/kg q 6 hr. *Bacteremia/meningitis* up to 75–100 mg/kg/day.

CNS: confusion, depression, headache.
EENT: blurred vision, optic neuritis.
GI: bitter taste (IV only); diarrhea, nausea, vomiting.
Derm: rashes.
Hemat: APLASTIC ANEMIA, bone marrow depression.
Neuro: peripheral neuritis.
Misc: GRAY SYNDROME in newborns, fever.

NOTES: **Contraindications:** Hypersensitivity, previous toxic reaction to chloramphenicol. **Cautions:** Newborns; patients with severe hepatic or renal disease; G6PD deficiency; porphyria; geriatric patients; pregnancy or lactation.

chloroquine *Anti-infective (antimalarial)* Pregnancy category UK	Prophylaxis and treatment of malaria; treatment of amebic liver abscess. **Unlabeled Uses:** Treatment of severe rheumatoid arthritis.	*Malaria* **PO (Adults):** *Suppression/chemoprophylaxis* 300 mg/week, starting 1–2 wk prior to entering malarious areas and for 4 wk afterward. *Treatment*—600 mg initially, then 300 mg at 6–8 hr, 24 hr, and 48 hr after initial dose (not to exceed 1 g/24 hr).

CNS: SEIZURES, anxiety, confusion, dizziness, fatigue, headache, irritability, personality changes.
EENT: keratopathy, ototoxicity; retinopathy, visual disturbances.
CV: ECG changes, hypotension.

(continued)

{ } available in Canada only. *CAPITALS indicate life-threatening, underlines indicate most frequent

P–139

ADDITIONAL DRUGS (CONTINUED)

Generic name Trade name(s) *Classification* Pregnancy category Scheduled substance	Indications	Adverse Reactions and Side Effects*	Route and Dosage
chloroquine (continued) *Anti-infective agents* *(antimalarial)* Pregnancy category UK	Doses expressed as chloroquine base: 1 mg of chloroquine base = 1.67 mg chloroquine phosphate or 1.25 mg chloroquine hydrochloride.	**GI:** abdominal cramps, anorexia, diarrhea, epigastric discomfort, nausea, vomiting. **GU:** discoloration of urine. **Derm:** alopecia, dermatoses, photosensitivity, pigmentary changes, pruritus, skin eruptions. **Hemat:** AGRANULOCYTOSIS, APLASTIC ANEMIA, LEUKOPENIA, thrombocytopenia. **Neuro:** neuromyopathy, peripheral neuritis.	***Malaria (continued)*** **PO (Children):** *Suppression/chemoprophylaxis* 5 mg/week, starting 1–2 wk prior to entering malarious areas and for 4 wk afterward (not to exceed 300 mg/day) *Treatment*—10 mg/kg initially, then 5 mg/kg at 6 hr, 24 hr, and 48 hr after initial dose (not to exceed 12.5 mg/kg/24 hr). **IM (Adults):** 160–200 mg, may repeat in 6 hr (not to exceed 800 mg/24 hr). **IM, SC (Children):** 3.5 mg/kg, may repeat in 6 hr (not to exceed 10 mg/kg/24 hr). **IV (Children):** 13.3 mg/kg initially, then 6.6 mg/kg q 6–8 hr. ***Amebic Liver Abscess*** **PO (Adults):** 150 mg 4 times daily for 2 days, then 150 mg twice daily for 2–3 wk (with other antiprotozoals). **PO (Children):** 6 mg/kg (up to 300 mg)/day for 3 wk. **IM (Adults):** 160–200 mg/day for 10-12 days. **IM (Children):** 6 mg/kg/day for 10-12 days. ***Rheumatoid Arthritis*** **PO (Adults):** Up to 2.4 mg/kg/day (based on ideal body weight).

NOTES: Contraindications: Hypersensitivity; hypersensitivity hydroxychloroquine; visual damage caused by chloroquine hydroxychloroquine. **Cautions:** Liver disease, alcoholism; patients receiving hepatotoxic drugs; porphyria; psoriasis; G6PD deficiency; bone marrow depression; pregnancy; lactation or children.

| clemastine
Antihist-1, Contac Allergy 12 Hour,
Tavist
Antihistamines
Pregnancy category B | Relief of allergic symptoms caused by histamine release including allergic rhinitis and urticaria. | **CNS:** drowsiness, confusion, dizziness, excitation (children).
EENT: blurred vision.
CV: hypertension, arrhythmias, hypotension, palpitations.
GI: dry mouth, constipation, obstruction.
GU: retention, hesitancy.
Derm: sweating. | **PO (Adults):** *Most allergic conditions* 1.34 mg twice daily. *Allergic dermatoses* 2.68 mg 1–3 times daily.
PO (Children 6-12 yr): *Most allergic conditions* 0.67 mg twice daily. *Allergic dermatoses* 1.34 mg twice daily (not to exceed 4.02 mg/day). |

NOTES: Cautions: Hypersensitivity; acute asthma; lactation; alcohol intolerance (liquid). **Use Cautiously in:** Glaucoma; liver disease; geriatric patients; pregnancy or children <6 yr.

clomiphene
Clomid, Milophene, Serophene
Hormones (ovulation inducers)
Pregnancy category X

Induces ovulation in anovulatory women who desire pregnancy. Requires intact anterior pituitary, thyroid, and adrenal function.
Unlabeled Uses: Male infertility due to oligospermia

CNS: fatigue, headache, insomnia, light-headedness, nervousness, restlessness.
EENT: blurred vision, photophobia, scotoma, visual disturbances.
CV: hot flashes, flushing.
GI: abdominal pain, bloating, distention, increased appetite, nausea, vomiting.
GU: increased urine volume, frequency.
Derm: allergic dermatitis, rashes, hair loss, urticaria.
Endo: cyst formation, ovarian enlargement, breast discomfort, multiple births.
Metab: weight gain.

PO (Adults): 25–50 mg/day for 5 days; if ovulation does not occur, a second course of 100 mg/day for 5 days may be given 30 days after the initial course. A maximum of 3 courses may be administered. Some patients require up to 250 mg/day.

NOTES: Contraindications: Liver disease, ovarian cysts, pregnancy. **Cautions:** Known sensitivity to pituitary gonadotropins, polycystic ovary syndrome.

---

dacarbazine
[DTIC]; DTIC-Dome
Antineoplastic agents (alkylating agents)
Pregnancy category C

Treatment of metastatic malignant melanoma (single agent).
Treatment of advanced Hodgkin's disease (with other agents).

GI: HEPATIC NECROSIS, anorexia, nausea, vomiting, diarrhea, hepatic vein thrombosis.
Derm: alopecia, facial flushing, photosensitivity.
Endo: gonadal suppression.
Hemat: bone marrow depression.
Local: pain at IV site, phlebitis at IV site, tissue necrosis.
MS: myalgia.
Neuro: facial paresthesia.
Misc: ANAPHYLAXIS, facial flushing, fever, flu-like syndrome, malaise.

IV (Adults): *Malignant melanoma*—2–4.5 mg/kg/day for 10 days q 4 wk *or* 250 mg/m^2/day for 5 days q 3 wk. *Hodgkin's disease*—150 mg/m^2/day for 5 days (in combination with other agents) q 4 wk *or* 375 mg/m^2 (with other agents) q 15 days.

NOTES: Contraindications: Hypersensitivity, pregnancy or lactation, concurrent radiation therapy. **Cautions:** Active infections, decreased bone marrow reserve, other chronic debilitating diseases, children, renal disease, patients with childbearing potential.

---

dactinomycin
actinomycin-D, Cosmegen
Antineoplastic agents (antitumor antibiotics)
Pregnancy category C

Used alone and in combination with other treatment modalities (other antineoplastic agents, radiation therapy, or surgery) in the management of Wilms' tumor, rhabdomyosarcoma, Ewing's sarcoma, trophoblastic neoplasms, testicular carcinoma, other malignancies.

CNS: lethargy, malaise.
GI: nausea, stomatitis, vomiting, hepatotoxicity, ulceration.
Derm: alopecia, photosensitivity, radiation recall, rashes.
Endo: gonadal suppression.
Hemat: anemia, leukopenia, thrombocytopenia.
Local: phlebitis at IV site.
Misc: fever.

IV (Adults): 10–15 mcg/kg/day for up to 5 days q 4-6 wk or 500 mcg/m^2 (up to 2 mg) weekly for 3 wk.
IV (Children >6 mo): 15 mcg/kg (450–500 mcg/m^2) daily for up to 5 days *or* 2.5 mg/m^2 total dose divided into 7 daily doses; may be repeated in 4–6 wk.

NOTES: Contraindications: Hypersensitivity, pregnant or lactating women. **Cautions:** Active infections; ↓ bone marrow reserve; concurrent radiation therapy; other chronic debilitating illnesses; obesity; patients with childbearing potential.

{ } available in Canada only. *CAPITALS indicate life-threatening, underlines indicate most frequent

ADDITIONAL DRUGS (CONTINUED)

Generic name Trade name(s) Classification Pregnancy category Scheduled substance	Indications	Adverse Reactions and Side Effects*	Route and Dosage
D-aminoglutethimide Cytadren *Antineoplastic agents* Pregnancy category D	Short-term adrenal suppression in patients with Cushing's syndrome. **Unlabeled use:** Metastatic breast or prostate cancer.	**CNS:** drowsiness, dizziness, headache, weakness. **CV:** hypotension. **GI:** anorexia, nausea, hepatitis, vomiting. **Derm:** measles-like rash, pruritus, urticaria. **Endo:** adrenal insufficiency/suppression, hypothyroidism, masculinization in women. **Hemat:** AGRANULOCYTOSIS, leukopenia, thrombocytopenia. **MS:** myalgia. **Misc:** fever.	***Cushing's Disease*** **PO (Adults):** 250 mg 2–3 times daily for 2 wk, then 250 mg q 6 hr (up to 2 g/day; mineralocorticoid supplements may be required). ***Breast or Prostate Cancer (unlabeled)*** **PO (Adults):** 125 mg twice daily for several days–1 wk, then 2–3 times daily for 2 wk, then 250 mg q 6 hr (up to 2 g/day; with hydrocortisone).

NOTES: Contraindications: Hypersensitivity to glutethimide/aminoglutethimide. **Cautions:** Stress; geriatric patients; renal impairment; pregnancy; lactation, or children.

Generic name	Indications	Adverse Reactions and Side Effects*	Route and Dosage
denileukin diftitox Ontak *Antineoplastic agents* *(cytotoxic protein)* Pregnancy category C	Persistent or recurrent cutaneous T-cell lymphoma whose malignant cells express the CD25 component of the interleukin-2 (IL-2) receptor.		**IV (Adults):** 9 or 18 mcg/kg/day for 5 days every 21 days.

NOTES: Contraindications: Hypersensitivity to denileukin, diphtheria toxin, or interleukin-2. **Cautions:** Geriatric patients, preexisting cardiovascular disease, pregnancy, or children.

Generic name	Indications	Adverse Reactions and Side Effects*	Route and Dosage
dextrose glucose, Glutose, Insta-glucose, Insulin Reaction *Nutritional products* *(carbohydrates)* Pregnancy category C	**IV:** Lower-concentration (2.5–11.5%) injection provides hydration and calories. Higher concentrations (up to 70%) treat hypoglycemia and in combination with amino acids provide calories for parenteral nutrition 50% treatment of hypoglycemia (hyperinsulinemia or insulin shock). **PO:** Corrects hypoglycemia in conscious patients.	**Endo:** inappropriate insulin secretion (long-term use). **F and E:** fluid overload, hypokalemia, hypomagnesemia, hypophosphatemia. **Local:** local pain and irritation at IV site (hypertonic solution). **Metab:** glycosuria, hyperglycemia.	***Hydration (as 5% solution)*** **IV (Adults and Children):** 0.5–0.8 g/kg/hr. ***Hypoglycemia*** **PO (Adults and Children):** *Conscious patients* 10–20 g, may repeat in 10–20 min. **IV (Adults):** 20–50 ml of 50% solution infused slowly (3 ml/min). **IV (Infants and Neonates):** 250–500 mg/kg/dose (as 25% dextrose); repeated doses of 10–12 ml of 25% dextrose may be required.

NOTES: Contraindications: Allergy to corn or corn products; hypertonic solution should not be given to patients with CNS bleeding; dehydration. **Use Cautiously in:** Diabetic patients; chronic alcoholic patients/severely malnourished patients.

dicyclomine
Bentyl, [Bentylol], (Formulex), (Spasmoban)
Anticholinergic agents (antispasmodics)
Pregnancy category UK

Management of irritable bowel syndrome in patients who do not respond to usual interventions (sedation/change in diet).

PO (Adults): 10–20 mg 3–4 times daily (up to 160 mg/day).
PO (Children 2 yr): 10 mg 3–4 times daily, adjusted as tolerated.
PO (Children 6 mo–2 yr): 5–10 mg 3–4 times daily, adjusted as tolerated.
IM (Adults): 20 mg q 4–6 hr, adjusted as tolerated.

CNS: confusion (increased in geriatric patients), drowsiness, light-headedness (IM only).
EENT: blurred vision, increased intraocular pressure.
CV: palpitations, tachycardia.
GI: PARALYTIC ILEUS, constipation, heartburn, decreased salivation, dry mouth, nausea, vomiting.
GU: impotence, urinary hesitancy, urinary retention.
Derm: decreased sweating.
Endo: decreased lactation.
Local: pain/redness at IM site.
Misc: allergic reactions including ANAPHYLAXIS.

NOTES: **Contraindications:** Hypersensitivity; obstruction of the GI/GU tract; reflux esophagitis; severe ulcerative colitis; unstable cardiovascular status; glaucoma; myasthenia gravis, infants <6 mo; lactation. Use **Cautiously in:** High environmental temperatures; hepatic/renal impairment, autonomic neuropathy, cardiovascular disease, prostatic hyperplasia, geriatric patients, pregnancy.

---

diflunisal
[Apo-Diflunisal], Dolobid, Novo-Diflunisal
Non-opioid analgesics
Nonsteroidal anti-inflammatory agents
Pregnancy category B, (C first trimester)

Inflammatory disorders including rheumatoid arthritis, osteoarthritis, and treatment of mild to moderate pain.

PO (Adults): *Anti-inflammatory*—250–500 mg twice daily. *Analgesic*—500 mg–1 g initially, then 250–500 mg q 8–12 hr.

CNS: dizziness, drowsiness, headache, psychic disturbances.
EENT: blurred vision, rhinitis, tinnitus.
CV: arrhythmias, changes in blood pressure, edema.
GI: GI BLEEDING, discomfort, nausea, constipation, diarrhea, vomiting.
GU: renal failure.
Derm: rashes.
Hemat: blood dyscrasias, prolonged bleeding time.
MS: muscle aches.
Misc: allergic reactions including ANAPHYLAXIS, chills.

NOTES: **Contraindications:** Hypersensitivity; cross-sensitivity may occur with other NSAIDs; active GI bleeding/ulcer disease. **Cautions:** Cardiovascular, renal/hepatic disease; history of ulcer disease; adolescents; pregnancy, lactation, or children.

---

edrophonium
Enlon, Reversol, Tensilon
Cholinergic agents (anticholinesterase)
Pregnancy category C

Diagnosis of myasthenia gravis. Assessment of adequacy of anticholin-esterase therapy in myasthenia gravis. Differentiating myasthenic from cholinergic crisis. Reversal of muscle paralysis from nondepolarizing neuromuscular blockers.

Diagnosis of Myasthenia Gravis
IV (Adults): 2 mg; if no response, may give 8 mg after 45 sec; may repeat test in 30 min. If cholinergic response occurs, administer atropine 0.4 mg IV. Patients >50 yr should be pretreated with atropine
IV (Children >34 kg): 2 mg; if no response after 45 sec, may give 1 mg q 30–45 sec to a total of 10 mg. If cholinergic response occurs, administer atropine IV.
IV (Children <34 kg): 1 mg; if no response after 45 sec, may give 1 mg q 45 sec to a total of 5 mg. If cholinergic response occurs, administer atropine IV.

CNS: SEIZURES, dizziness, weakness.
EENT: lacrimation, miosis.
Resp: bronchospasm, excess secretions.
CV: bradycardia, hypotension.
GI: abdominal cramps, diarrhea, excess salivation, vomiting, nausea.
Derm: sweating, rashes.
MS: fasciculation.

(continued)

[ ] available in Canada only. *CAPITALS indicate life-threatening, underlines indicate most frequent

ADDITIONAL DRUGS (CONTINUED)

Generic name Trade name(s) *Classification* Pregnancy category Scheduled substance	Indications	Adverse Reactions and Side Effects*	Route and Dosage
edrophonium (continued) Enlon, Reversol, Tensilon *Cholinergic agents* *(anticholinesterase)* Pregnancy category C			***Diagnosis of Myasthenia Gravis (continued)*** **IV (Infants):** 0.5 mg. **IM (Adults):** 10 mg. If cholinergic response occurs, may repeat 2-mg dose in 30 min to rule out false-negative reaction. Patients >50 yr should be pretreated with atropine. **IM (Children >34 kg):** 5 mg. **IM (Children <34 kg):** 2 mg. ***Assessment of Anticholinesterase Therapy*** **IV (Adults):** 1–2 mg 1 hr after oral anticholinesterase. ***Differentiation of Cholinergic from Myasthenic Crisis*** **IV (Adults):** 1 mg; may give additional 1 mg 1 min later. ***Reversal of Nondepolarizing Neuromuscular Blocking Agents*** **IV (Adults):** 10 mg; repeat as needed (not to exceed 40 mg; range 0.5–1 mg/kg.

NOTES: Contraindications: Hypersensitivity; mechanical obstruction of the GI; GI tract; hypersensitivity to bisulfites; pregnancy; lactation. **Cautions:** Asthma or ulcer disease; cardiovascular disease; epilepsy; Hyperthyroidism. Atropine should be available in case of excessive dosage.

estramustine Emcyt *Antineoplastic agents* *(hormone/alkylating agents)* Pregnancy category UK	Palliative treatment of advanced metastatic prostate cancer.	**CNS:** insomnia. **CV:** THROMBOEMBOLISM, edema, hypertension. **GI:** diarrhea, nausea, vomiting. **Derm:** rashes. **Endo:** decreased libido, gynecomastia, gonadal suppression (azoospermia), hyperglycemia. **F and E:** sodium and water retention. **Hemat:** anemia, leukopenia, thrombocytopenia. **Misc:** allergic reactions, fever.	**PO (Adults):** 600 mg/m²/day in 3 divided doses *or* 14 mg/kg/day (range 10–16 mg/kg) in 3–4 divided doses.

NOTES: Contraindications: Thromboembolism/stroke/myocardial infarction; cross-sensitivity/tolerance to estradiol or mechlorethamine may occur. **Cautions:** Thromboembolic disorders; hypercalcemia; peptic ulcer; infection; renal / hepatic impairment; gallbladder disease; migraine headaches; metabolic bone disease; epilepsy; asthma; bone marrow depression; childbearing potential.

factor IX, human
AlphaNine SD, Benefix, Hemonyne, Konyne 80, Mononine, Profilnine SD, Proplex T

Hemostatic agents
(clotting factor)
Pregnancy category C

Treatment of active or impending bleeding due to factor IX deficiency (hemophilia B, Christmas disease).

Treatment of bleeding in patients with factor VIII inhibitors.

Prevention and treatment of bleeding in patients with factor VII deficiency (Proplex T only).

CNS: drowsiness, headache, lethargy.
CV: changes in blood pressure, changes in heart rate.
GI: nausea, vomiting.
Derm: flushing, urticaria.
Hemat: disseminated intravascular coagulation, thrombosis.
Neuro: tingling.
Misc: chills, fever, risk of transmission of viral hepatitis, risk of transmission of HIV virus, hypersensitivity reactions.

The following general formula may be used:
Human-derived products—Dose (units) = body weight (kg) × 1 unit/kg × desired factor IX increase (% of normal).
Recombinant DNA product—Dose (units) = body weight (kg) × 1.2 units/kg × desired factor IX increase (% of normal). Pre- and postoperatively maintain levels of >25% for at least 7 days. Calculate doses to ↑ levels to 40–60% of normal. High levels may require daily or twice-daily dosing, whereas q 2–3 day dosing will maintain lower levels. A single dose may stop a minor bleed.

NOTES: Contraindications: Factor VII deficiency (except Proplex T); intravascular coagulation or fibrinolysis associated with liver disease; allergy to mouse protein (Mononine). **Cautions:** Postoperative period (increased risk of thrombosis); blood groups A, B, or AB.

---

fenoprofen
Nalfon

Non-opioid analgesics
Nonsteroidal anti-inflammatory agents
Pregnancy Category B (first trimester)

Rheumatoid arthritis, osteoarthritis, and mild to moderate pain, including dysmenorrhea.

CNS: drowsiness, headache, dizziness, psychic disturbances.
EENT: blurred vision, tinnitus.
CV: arrhythmias, edema.
GI: GI BLEEDING, HEPATITIS, constipation, dyspepsia, nausea, vomiting, discomfort.
GU: cystitis, hematuria, renal failure.
Derm: rashes.
Hemat: blood dyscrasias, prolonged bleeding time.
Misc: allergic reactions including ANAPHYLAXIS.

Anti-inflammatory
PO (Adults): 300–600 mg 3–4 times daily (not to exceed 3.2 g/day).
Analgesic
PO (Adults): 200 mg q 4–6 hr.

NOTES: Contraindications: Hypersensitivity; cross-sensitivity may occur with other NSAIDs; active GI bleeding/ulcer disease. **Cautions:** Severe cardiovascular/renal/hepatic disease; history of ulcer disease; pregnancy, lactation, or children.

---

fluoride (topical)
ACT, Fluorigard, Fluorinse, Gel Kam, Gel-Tin, Karigel, Listermint with Fluoride, Minute-Gel, MouthKote F/R, Point Two, Stop, Thera-Flu

Dental caries prophylactic agents
Mineral supplements
Pregnancy category UK

Prevention of dental caries in children where insufficient fluoride is available in drinking water.

CNS: headache, weakness.
GI: gastric distress.
Derm: atopic dermatitis, eczema, urticaria.
Misc: mottling of teeth (toxicity).

Topical (Adults and Children >12 yr): 10 ml/day. (Point Two is used once weekly.)
Topical (Children 6–12 yr): 5–10 ml/day. (Point Two is used once weekly.)

NOTES: Contraindications: Hypersensitivity; where fluoride in drinking water exceeds 0.7 parts per million (ppm); some products contain tartrazine or alcohol and should be avoided in patients ith known intolerance, severe renal impairment. **Cautions:** Situations where fluoride content of water is unknown.

( ) available in Canada only. *CAPITALS indicate life-threatening, underlines indicate most frequent

ADDITIONAL DRUGS (CONTINUED)

Generic name Trade name(s) *Classification* Pregnancy category Scheduled substance	Indications	Adverse Reactions and Side Effects*	Route and Dosage
gold sodium thiomalate Aurolate, Aurothioglucose *Antirheumatic agents (disease-modifying)* Pregnancy category C	Treatment of progressive rheumatoid arthritis resistant to conventional therapy.	**CNS:** dizziness, headache, syncope. **EENT:** corneal gold deposits, corneal ulcerations. **Resp:** pneumonitis. **CV:** bradycardia. **GI:** abdominal pain, cramping, diarrhea, metallic taste, stomatitis, anorexia, dysphagia, hepatitis, dyspepsia, flatulence, nausea, vomiting. **Derm:** dermatitis, rash, photosensitivity, pruritus. **Hemat:** AGRANULOCYTOSIS, APLASTIC ANEMIA, thrombocytopenia, eosinophilia, leukopenia. **Neuro:** neuropathy. **Misc:** allergic reactions, including ANAPHYLAXIS, angioneurotic edema, nitritoid reactions.	**IM (Adults):** 10 mg initially, then 25 mg 1 wk later, followed by 25–50 mg weekly until improvement or toxicity occurs, up to 1 g total, then 25–50 mg q 2 wk for up to 20 wk, then q 3–4 wk. *History of a previous mild reaction*—Reinstitute with an initial dose of 5 mg, increasing by 5–10 mg weekly or monthly until a dose of 25–50 mg is reached. **IM (Children):** 10 mg initially, followed 1 wk later by 1 mg/kg q 2 wk for up to 20 wk, then q 3–4 wk.

NOTES: Contraindication: Hypersensitivity; severe hepatic/renal dysfunction; previous heavy metal toxicity; history of colitis or exfoliative dermatitis; uncontrolled diabetes; tuberculosis; CHF; Systemic lupus erythematosus; recent radiation therapy; debilitated patients; pregnancy or lactation. **Cautions:** History of blood dyscrasias: hypertension; rashes.

hetastarch Hespan *Volume expanders* Pregnancy category C	Adjunct for fluid replacement and volume expansion in the early management of shock or impending shock caused by: burns, hemorrhage, surgery, sepsis or trauma. Adjunct in leukapheresis (improves collection of granulocytes).	**CNS:** headache. **CV:** CHF, pulmonary edema. **GI:** vomiting. **Derm:** pruritus, urticaria. **F and E:** fluid overload, lower extremity edema **Hemat:** ↓hematocrit, ↓ platelet function. **MS:** myalgia. **Misc:** hypersensitivity reactions including ANAPHYLACTOID REACTIONS, chills, fever, paroid/submaxillary gland enlargement.	**IV (Adults):** 30–60 g (500–1000 ml of 6% solution), may be repeated; not to exceed 90 g (1500 ml/day). In acute hemorrhagic shock, up to 20 ml/kg/hr may be used.

NOTES: Contraindications: Hypersensitivity, severe bleeding disorders, CHF, pulmonary edema, oliguric or anuric renal failure, early pregnancy. **Cautions:** Thrombocytopenia, severe renal impairment; geriatric patients, lactation, or children (safety not established).

immune globulin IM Gamastan, IGIM, Gammar		**CNS:** faintness, headache, light-headedness, malaise. **Resp:** dyspnea, wheezing.	

Drug	Action/Uses	Side effects/Adverse reactions	Dosage
Anti-infective agents (immune globulin) Pregnancy category UK	Provides passive immunity to a variety of infections including: hepatitis A and measles (rubeola) when immune sera are unavailable or when there is insufficient time for active immunization to take place	**CV:** chest pain. **GI:** nausea. **GU:** RENAL FAILURE, diuresis (if maltose in preparation), nephrotic syndrome. **Derm:** cyanosis, urticaria. **Local:** muscle stiffness, pain, tenderness. **MS:** arthralgia, back pain, hip pain. **Misc:** allergic reactions including ANAPHYLAXIS, angioedema, chills, fever, sweating.	***Hepatitis A Prophylaxis*** **IM (Adults and Children):** 0.02 ml/kg (for pre-exposure prophylaxis, higher doses 0.06 ml/kg q 4–6 mo are used if exposure will last >3 mo). ***Measles Prophylaxis*** **IM (Adults and Children):** 0.25 ml/kg (0.5 ml/kg if immunosuppressed; not to exceed 15 ml).

NOTES: Contraindications: Hypersensitivity to immune globulins or additives; selective IgA deficiency. **Cautions:** Thrombocytopenia; has been used during pregnancy, although safety is not established.

Drug	Action/Uses	Side effects/Adverse reactions	Dosage
immune globulin IV Gamimune N, Gammagard S/D, Gammar-P IV, IG IV, Iveegam, Polygam, Polygam S/D, Sandoglobulin, Venoglobulin-I, Venoglobulin-S *Anti-infective agents (immune globulins)* Pregnancy Category UK	Useful in patients with immunodeficiency syndromes who are unable to produce IgG-type antibodies. Prevention of bacterial infections in patients with B-cell chronic lymphocytic leukemia (Gammagard only). Prevention of bacterial infections in children infected with HIV; treatment of idiopathic thrombocytopenic purpura. Treatment of Kawasaki syndrome (Iveegam and Gammagard SD)	**CNS:** faintness, headache, light-headedness, malaise. **Resp:** dyspnea, wheezing. **CV:** chest pain. **GI:** nausea. **GU:** RENAL FAILURE, diuresis (if maltose in preparation), nephrotic syndrome. **Derm:** cyanosis, urticaria. **Local:** *at IM site*—muscle stiffness, pain, tenderness; *at IV site*—local inflammation, phlebitis. **MS:** arthralgia, back pain, hip pain. **Misc:** allergic reactions including ANAPHYLAXIS, angioedema, chills, fever, sweating.	***Immunodeficiency*** **IV (Adults and Children):** 100–800 mg/kg q 3–4 wk (other regimens are used). ***Idiopathic Thrombocytopenic Purpura*** **IV (Adults and Children):** 400 mg/kg/day for 5 days; maybe be repeated (other regimens are used). ***Prevention of Bacterial Infections in HIV-Infected Patients*** **IV (Adults and Children):** 400 mg/kg q 3–4 wk. ***Kawasaki Syndrome*** **IV (Children):** 400 mg/kg/day for 4 consecutive days or 1 g/kg single dose over 10 hr (Iveegam) given with aspirin therapy; must be started within 10 days of onset of symptoms.

NOTES: Contraindication: Hypersensitivity to immune globulins or additives; selective IgA deficiency. **Cautions:** Gamimune N product in patients with acid-base disorders; products containing sucrose (may have increased risk of renal failure (Sandoglobulin, Gammar P IV, Gammar IV); agammaglobulinemia or hypogammaglobulinemia. Has been used during pregnancy, although safety is not established.

Drug	Action/Uses	Side effects/Adverse reactions	Dosage
interferon alfa-2a, recombinant Roferon-A *Antineoplastic agents Immune modifiers* Pregnancy category C	Treatment of Hairy cell leukemia, AIDS-associated Kaposi's sarcoma, chronic myelogenous leukemia	**CNS:** depression with suicidal ideation, dizziness, confusion, insomnia, nervousness, trouble concentrating, trouble thinking. **EENT:** blurred vision. **CV:** arrhythmias, chest pain. **GI:** anorexia, decreased appetite, diarrhea, dry mouth, nausea, stomatitis, taste disorder, vomiting, weight loss, drug-induced hepatitis (↑ in Kaposi's sarcoma). **GU:** gonadal suppression.	**IM, SC (Adults):** *Hairy cell leukemia (induction)* —3 million units/day for 16–24 wk. If severe adverse reactions occur, reduce dosage by 50%. *Hairy cell leukemia (maintenance)* —3 million units 3 times weekly. *Kaposi's sarcoma (induction)* —36 million units/day for 10–12 wk or 3 million units/day for 3 days, then 9 million units/day for next 3 days, then 18 million units/day for next 3 days, then 36 million units/day for rest of 10–12 wk course.

(continued)

{ } available in Canada only. *CAPITALS indicate life-threatening, underlines indicate most frequent

ADDITIONAL DRUGS (CONTINUED)

Generic name Trade name(s) *Classification* Pregnancy category Scheduled substance	Indications	Adverse Reactions and Side Effects[a]	Route and Dosage
interferon alfa-2a, recombinant (continued) Roferon-A *Antineoplastic agents* *Immune modifiers* Pregnancy category C		**Derm:** pruritus, rash, alopecia, dry skin, sweating. **Endo:** thyroid disorders (↑ in Kaposi's sarcoma). **Hemat:** anemia, leukopenia, thrombocytopenia. **MS:** leg cramps. **Neuro:** peripheral neuropathy. **Misc:** chills, fever, flu-like syndrome.	*Kaposi's sarcoma (maintenance)*—36 million units 3 times weekly. *Chronic myelogenous leukemia*—9 million units/day (may be started as 3 million units/day for 3 days, then 6 million units/day for 3 days, then 9 million units/day).
NOTES: **Contraindications:** Hypersensitivity to alfa interferons, human serum albumin, or mouse immunoglobulin. **Cautions:** Severe cardiovascular, pulmonary, renal, or hepatic disease; infections; underlying CNS pathology/psychiatric history; decreased bone marrow reserve/underlying immunosuppression; current history of chickenpox; herpes zoster, or herpes; previous or concurrent radiation therapy; geriatric/debilitated patients; history of suicide attempt; childbearing potential; lactation and children <18 yr (safety not established).			
interferon alfa-2b, recombinant Intron A *Antineoplastic agents* *Immune modifiers* Pregnancy category C	Treatment of: Hairy cell leukemia, malignant melanoma, AIDS-associated Kaposi's sarcoma, condyloma acuminatum (intralesional), chronic hepatitis non-A, non-B/C infection, chronic hepatitis B infection. Treatment of chronic hepatitis C infection (with oral ribavirin) that has relapsed following previous treatment with[‡] interferon alone.	**CNS:** dizziness, confusion, depression with suicidal ideation, insomnia, nervousness, trouble concentrating, trouble thinking. **EENT:** blurred vision. **CV:** arrhythmias, chest pain. **GI:** anorexia, decreased appetite, diarrhea, dry mouth, nausea, stomatitis, taste disorder, vomiting, weight loss, drug-induced hepatitis (increased in Kaposi's sarcoma). **GU:** gonadal suppression. **Derm:** pruritus, rash, alopecia, dry skin, sweating. **Endo:** thyroid disorders (increased in Kaposi's sarcoma). **Hemat:** anemia, leukopenia, thrombocytopenia. **MS:** leg cramps. **Neuro:** peripheral neuropathy. **Misc:** chills, fever, flu-like syndrome.	**IV (Adults):** *Malignant melanoma*—20 million units/m²/day for 5 days of each week for 4 wk initially, followed by SC maintenance dosing. **IM, SC (Adults):** *Hairy cell leukemia*—2 million units/m² 3 times weekly. *Malignant melanoma*—10 million units/m²/day 3 times weekly for 48 wk, following initial IV dosing. *Kaposi's sarcoma*—30 million units/m² 3 times weekly. *Chronic hepatitis non-A/non-B/C infection*—3 million units 3 times weekly for 24 mo (if relapse occurs, oral ribavarin may be added). *Chronic hepatitis B infection*—5 million units/day or 10 million units 3 times weekly for 16 wk. **IL (Adults):** *Condyloma acuminatum*—1 million units/lesion 3 times weekly for 3 wk; treat only 5 lesions per course.
NOTES: **Contraindications:** Hypersensitivity to alfa interferons or human serum albumin. **Cautions:** Severe cardiovascular/pulmonary/renal/hepatic disease; infections; CNS pathology/psychiatric history; ↓ bone marrow reserve/underlying immunosuppression; current history of chickenpox, herpes zoster, or herpes labialis; history of radiation therapy; geriatric/debilitated patients; history of suicide attempt; patients with childbearing potential; lactation, and children <18			

interferon alfa-n3, human Alferon N *Antineoplastic agents* *Immune modifiers* *Pregnancy category C*	Treatment of condyloma acuminatum (intralesional).	**IL (Adults):** 250,000 units/lesion twice weekly for up to 8 wk; for large lesions, divide dose and inject at several sites.
CNS: dizziness. **MS:** myalgias. **Misc:** flu-like symptoms.		

NOTES: Contraindications: Hypersensitivity to human alfa interferons, mouse immunoglobulin, neomycin, or egg protein. **Cautions:** Debilitating medical conditions; coagulation disorders; pregnancy, lactation, or children.

lepirudin (rDNA) Refludan *Anticoagulants (thrombin inhibitors)* *Pregnancy category B*	Management of thromboembolic disease and prevention of its complications in patients who have experienced heparin-induced thrombocytopenia.	**IV (Adults):** 0.4 mg/kg (not to exceed 44 mg) as a bolus over 15–20 sec, followed by 0.15 mg/kg/hr (not to exceed 16.5 mg/hr) initially, further adjustments made on the basis of laboratory assessment (aPTT) but should not exceed infusion rate of 0.21 mg/kg/hr without checking for coagulation abnormalities
Hemat: bleeding. **Misc:** allergic reactions: including ANAPHYLAXIS.		

NOTES: Contraindications: Hypersensitivity; severe renal impairment. **Cautions:** Recent puncture of large vessels/organ biopsy; vessel/organ anomaly; recent CVA, stroke, intracerebral surgery or other neuroaxial procedure; severe uncontrolled hypertension; bacterial endocarditis; bleeding diatheses; recent major surgery; recent major bleeding; severe liver disease; moderate renal impairment; pregnancy, lactation or children.

levetiracetam Keppra *Anticonvulsants* *Pregnancy category C*	Adjunctive therapy in the treatment of partial onset seizures in adults.	**PO (Adults):** 500 mg twice daily initially; may be increased by 1000 mg/day at 2 wk intervals up to 3000 mg/day; *CCr 5–80 ml/min:* 500–1000 mg q 12 hr initially; *CCr 30–50 ml/min:* 250–750 mg q 12 hr initially; *CCr <30 ml/min:* 250–500 mg q 12 hr initially.
CNS: drowsiness, weakness. **Neuro:** coordination difficulties.		

NOTES: Contraindications: Hypersensitivity. **Cautions:** Geriatric patients; renal impairment.

levorphanol Levo-Dromoran, Levorphan *Opioid analgesics (agonist)* *Schedule II* *Pregnancy Category C*	Moderate to severe pain.	**PO (Adults 50 kg):** *Initial dosing in opioid-naive patients*—4 mg q 6–8 hr. **PO (Adults and Children <50 kg):** *Initial dosing in opioid-naive patients* 0.04 mg/kg q 6–8 hr (unlabeled for use in children). **SC, IV (Adults 50 kg):** *Initial dosing in opioid-naive patients*—2 mg q 6–8 hr. *Preoperative use*—1–2 mg SC 90 min before procedure. **SC, IV (Adults and Children <50 kg):** *Initial dosing in opioid-naive patients*—0.02 mg/kg q 6–8 hr (unlabeled for use in children).
CNS: confusion, sedation, dysphoria, euphoria, floating feeling, hallucinations, headache, unusual dreams. **EENT:** blurred vision, diplopia, miosis. **Resp:** respiratory depression. **CV:** hypotension, bradycardia. **GI:** constipation, dry mouth, nausea, vomiting. **GU:** urinary retention. **Derm:** flushing, sweating. **Misc:** physical dependence, psychological dependence, tolerance.		

NOTES: Contraindications: Hypersensitivity; avoid chronic use during pregnancy or lactation. **Cautions:** Head trauma, increased intracranial pressure; severe renal/hepatic/pulmonary disease; hypothyroidism; adrenal insufficiency; alcoholism; undiagnosed abdominal pain; prostatic hypertrophy; geriatric/debilitated patients. Larger doses may be required during chronic use.

{} available in Canada only. *CAPITALS indicate life-threatening, underlines indicate most frequent

ADDITIONAL DRUGS (CONTINUED)

Generic name Trade name(s) *Classification* Pregnancy category Scheduled substance	Indications	Adverse Reactions and Side Effects*	Route and Dosage
lomustine CCNU, CeeNu *Antineoplastic agents (nitrosurea)* Pregnancy category D	Alone or with other treatment modalities in the management of primary and metastatic brain tumors and Hodgkin's disease. **Unlabeled uses:** Bronchogenic carcinoma, non-Hodgkin's lymphoma, malignant melanoma, breast carcinoma, renal cell carcinoma, GI tract carcinoma.	**CNS:** ataxia, disorientation, dysarthria, lethargy. **Resp:** fibrosis, pulmonary infiltrates. **GI:** nausea, vomiting, anorexia, hepatotoxicity, stomatitis. **GU:** azotemia, renal failure. **Endo:** infertility. **Hemat:** leukopenia, thrombocytopenia, anemia. **Metab:** hyperuricemia. **Misc:** secondary malignancy (long-term use).	**PO (Adults and Children):** 100–130 mg/m² as a single dose every 6 wk. Dosage adjustments are required for concurrent therapy or decreased blood counts.

NOTES: Contraindications: Hypersensitivity; pregnancy or lactation. **Cautions:** Patients with childbearing potential; infections; decreased bone marrow reserve; geriatric/ debilitated patients; impaired liver function.

loxapine [Loxapac], Loxitane, Loxitane C, Loxitane IM *Antipsychotic agents* Pregnancy category C	Psychoses. **Unlabeled Uses:** Depression and anxiety associated with depression	**CNS:** NEUROLEPTIC MALIGNANT SYNDROME, confusion, dizziness, drowsiness, extrapyramidal reactions, headache, insomnia, syncope, tardive dyskinesia, weakness. **EENT:** blurred vision, lens opacities, nasal congestion. **CV:** orthostatic hypotension, tachycardia. **GI:** constipation, hepatitis, dry mouth, ileus, nausea, vomiting. **GU:** urinary retention. **Derm:** dermatitis, edema, photosensitivity, pigment changes, rashes, seborrhea. **Endo:** galactorrhea. **Hemat:** AGRANULOCYTOSIS. **Neuro:** ataxia. **Misc:** allergic reactions.	**PO (Adults):** 10 mg bid, may be increased gradually over the first 7–10 days as needed and tolerated. Usual maintenance dose is 15–25 mg 2–4 times daily. Severely ill patients may require up to 50 mg/day initially and maintenance doses up to 250 mg/day. **IM (Adults):** 12.5–50 mg q 4–6 hr as needed and tolerated (up to 250 mg/day).

NOTES: Contraindications: Hypersensitivity or intolerance to loxapine or amoxapine; coma; CNS depression; pregnancy or lactation. **Use Cautiously in:** Glaucoma; intestinal obstruction; epilepsy; alcoholism; cardiovascular disease; impaired liver function; geriatric patients (more susceptible to adverse reactions); children <16 yr.

mesoridazine Serentil	Acute and chronic psychoses.	**CNS:** NEUROLEPTIC MALIGNANT SYNDROME, drowsiness, extrapyramidal reactions, tardive dyskinesia.	**PO (Adults and Children >12 yr):** 30–150 mg/day in 2–3 divided doses.

| *Antipsychotic agents (phenothiazine)* Pregnancy category C | | **EENT:** blurred vision, dry eyes, lens opacities. **CV:** hypotension, tachycardia. **GI:** constipation, dry mouth, anorexia, ileus, drug-induced hepatitis. **GU:** urinary retention. **Derm:** photosensitivity, pigment changes, rashes. **Endo:** galactorrhea. **Hemat:** AGRANULOCYTOSIS, leukopenia. **Misc:** allergic reactions, hyperthermia. | **IM (Adults):** 25 mg; may be repeated in 30–60 min if needed and tolerated (range 25–200 mg/day). |

NOTES: **Contraindications:** Hypersensitivity, cross-sensitivity with other phenothiazines may occur; glaucoma; bone marrow depression; severe liver/cardiovascular disease; known alcohol intolerance (oral concentrate only). Use **Cautiously in:** Geriatric/emaciated/debilitated patients; diabetes; prostatic hypertrophy; CNS tumors; epilepsy; intestinal obstruction; pregnancy or lactation. **Interactions:** ↑ hypotension with acute ingestion of alcohol, antihypertensives or nitrates. Additive CNS depression with other CNS depressants. Concurrent use with lithium may produce any of the following: ↓ absorption, ↑ excretion of lithium, ↑ risk of extrapyramidal reactions, or masking of the early signs of lithium toxicity. Antacids/adsorbent antidiarrheals may ↓ absorption. ↑ risk of agranulocytosis with antithyroid drugs. May ↓ antiparkinson activity of levodopa and bromocriptine. ↓ vasopressor response to epinephrine and norepinephrine. ↓ antihypertensive effect of guanethidine. Concurrent use with beta blockers may result in inhibition of metabolism of one or both drugs, producing an ↑ response. ↑ risk of anticholinergic effects with other agents having anticholinergic properties.

| **mezlocillin** Anti-infective agents (extended–spectrum penicillin) Pregnancy category B | Treatment of serious infections due to susceptible organisms, including skin and skin structure infections, bone and joint infections, septicemia, respiratory tract infections, intra-abdominal, gynecologic, and urinary tract infections. Combination with an aminoglycoside may be synergistic against *Pseudomonas*. Has been combined with other antibiotics in the treatment of infections in immunosuppressed patients. | **CNS:** SEIZURES (high doses), confusion, lethargy. **CV:** ARRHYTHMIAS, CONGESTIVE HEART FAILURE. **GI:** PSEUDOMEMBRANOUS COLITIS, diarrhea, nausea. **GU:** hematuria (children). **Derm:** rashes, urticaria. **F and E:** hypokalemia, hypernatremia. **Hemat:** bleeding, blood dyscrasias. **Local:** pain at IM site, phlebitis at IV site. **Metab:** metabolic alkalosis. **Misc:** hypersensitivity reactions including ANAPHYLAXIS and SERUM SICKNESS, superinfection. | **IV, IM (Adults):** *Most infections*—3–4 g q 4–6 hr or 500 mg/kg q 8 hr IV (up to 24 g/day). *Complicated urinary tract infections*—3 g q 6 hr. *Uncomplicated urinary tract infections* 1.5 2 g q 6 hr. **IM, IV (Children 1 mo–12 yr):** 50 mg/kg q 4 hr. **IM, IV (Neonates 2 kg):** 50 mg/kg q 8 hr for the first 7 days of life, then increase to 50 mg/kg q 6 hr. **IM, IV (Neonates <2 kg):** 50 75 mg/kg q 12 hr for the first 7 days of life, then increase to 50 mg/kg q 8 hr. *Renal Impairment* **IM, IV (Adults):** *CCr 10–30 ml/min* 1.5–3 g q 6–8 hr; *CCr <10 ml/min* 1.5–2 g q 8 hr. |

NOTES: **Contraindications:** Hypersensitivity to penicillins. **Cautions:** Hypersensitivity to cephalosporins; severe renal/liver impairment; pregnancy and lactation.

| **mineral oil** Agoral, Fleet Mineral Oil, {Kondremul}, Kondremul Plain, {Lansoyl}, Liqui-Doss, Milkinol, Neo-Cultol, Nujol, Petrogalar Plain, Zymenol *Laxatives (lubricants)* Pregnancy category UK | Used to soften impacted feces in the management of constipation. | **Resp:** lipid pneumonia. **GI:** anal irritation, rectal seepage of mineral oil. | **PO (Adults and Children >12 yr):** 5–45 ml. **PO (Children 6–12 yr):** 5–20 ml. **Rect (Adults and Children >12 yr):** 60–150 ml as a single dose. **Rect (Children 2–11 yr):** 30–60 ml as a single dose. |

NOTES: **Contraindications:** Hypersensitivity; children <6 yr (oral); children <2 yr (rect). **Cautions:** Children, geriatric, or debilitated patients; pregnancy (may cause hypoprothrombinemia in newborn).

{} available in Canada only. *CAPITALS indicate life-threatening, underlines indicate most frequent

ADDITIONAL DRUGS (CONTINUED)

Generic name	Indications	Adverse Reactions and Side Effects*	Route and Dosage
Trade name(s)			
Classification			
Pregnancy category			
Scheduled substance			
multiple vitamins (intravenous): B complex with C and B, Cernevit-12, Multi Vitamin Concentrate, M.V.I.-12, M.V.I. Pediatric Vitamins (multiple, parenteral) Pregnancy category K	**IV:** Treatment and prevention of vitamin deficiencies in patients who are unable to ingest oral feedings or vitamins. **PO:** Treatment and prevention of vitamin deficiencies. Special formulations are available for patients with particular needs, including prenatal multiple vitamins (with larger doses of folic acid), preconceptional multiple vitamins, multiple vitamins with iron, multiple vitamins with fluoride, multiple vitamins with other minerals or trace elements.	**Misc:** allergic reactions to preservatives, additives, or colorants. In recommended doses, adverse reactions are extremely rare.	**IV (Adults and Children):** Amount sufficient to meet RDA (Recommended Daily Allowances) for age group. Usually added to large-volume parenteral or total parenteral nutrition (hyperalimentation) solution. **PO (Adults and Children):** 1 dosage unit (tablet/capsule/dropperful)/day or amount recommended by individual manufacturer.
multiple vitamins (oral): Adavite, Certagen, Dayalets, Hexavitamin, LKV Drops, Multi-75, Multi-Day, Nu-trox, One-A-Day, Optilets, Poly-Vi-Sol, Quintabs, Rulets, Sesame Street Vitamins, Sigtab, Stuyrite, Tab-A-Vite, Therabid, Theragran, Thera Multi-Vitamin, Theravee, Theravim, Theravite, Therems, Unicaps, Vita-Bob, Vita-Kid, Zymacap Vitamins (multiple, oral) Pregnancy category K			

NOTES: Hypersensitivity to preservatives, colorants, or additives, including tartrazine, saccharin, and aspartame (oral forms). Some products contain alcohol and should be avoided in patients with known intolerance. **Use Cautiously in:** Patients with anemia of undetermined cause. Large amounts of vitamin B₆ may interfere with the beneficial effect of levodopa.

| olsalazine Dipentum Anti-inflammatory agents (gastrointestinal/local) Pregnancy category C | Management of ulcerative colitis in patients who cannot tolerate sulfasalazine | **CNS:** ataxia, confusion, dizziness, drowsiness, headache, mental depression, psychosis, restlessness. **GI:** diarrhea, abdominal pain, anorexia, exacerbation of colitis, drug-induced hepatitis, nausea, vomiting. **Derm:** itching, rash. **Hemat:** blood dyscrasias. | **PO (Adults):** 500 mg twice daily. |

NOTES: **Contraindications:** Hypersensitivity reactions to salicylates (cross-sensitivity with furosemide, sulfonylurea hypoglycemic agents, or carbonic anhydrase inhibitors may occur); G6PD deficiency; urinary tract/ intestinal obstruction; porphyria; children <2 yr. **Cautions:** Severe hepatic/renal impairment; pregnancy; lactation.

Drug	Uses	Side effects	Dosage
oxymorphone Numorphan *Opioid analgesics (agonists)* Schedule II Pregnancy Category UK	Management of moderate to severe pain. Supplement in balanced anesthesia.	**CNS:** confusion, sedation, dizziness, dysphoria, euphoria, floating feeling, hallucinations, headache, unusual dreams. **EENT:** blurred vision, diplopia, miosis. **Resp:** RESPIRATORY DEPRESSION. **CV:** orthostatic hypotension. **GI:** constipation, dry mouth, nausea, vomiting. **GU:** urinary retention. **Derm:** flushing, sweating. **Misc:** physical dependence, psychological dependence, tolerance.	Larger doses may be required during chronic therapy. **SC, IM (Adults):** 1–1.5 mg q 3–6 hr as needed. *Analgesia during labor*—0.5–1 mg. **IV (Adults):** 0.5 mg q 3–6 hr as needed; increase as needed. **Rect (Adults):** 5 mg q 4–6 hr as needed.

NOTES: **Contraindications:** Hypersensitivity; avoid chronic use during pregnancy or lactation; children <12 yr. **Cautions:** Head trauma; increased intracranial pressure; severe renal/hepatic/pulmonary disease; hypothyroidism; adrenal insufficiency; alcoholism; geriatric/debilitated patients; undiagnosed abdominal pain; prostatic hypertrophy.

Drug	Uses	Side effects	Dosage
perphenazine (Apo-Perphenazine), PMS Perphenazine), Trilafon *Antipsychotic agents* *Antiemetic agents (phenothiazine)* Pregnancy category C	Acute and chronic psychoses, nausea, vomiting, or intractable hiccups.	**CNS:** NEUROLEPTIC MALIGNANT SYNDROME, extrapyramidal reactions, sedation, tardive dyskinesia. **EENT:** blurred vision, dry eyes, lens opacities. **CV:** hypotension, tachycardia. **GI:** constipation, dry mouth, anorexia, drug-induced hepatitis, ileus. **GU:** discoloration of urine, urinary retention. **Derm:** photosensitivity, pigment changes, rashes. **Endo:** galactorrhea. **Hemat:** AGRANULOCYTOSIS, leukopenia. **Metab:** hyperthermia. **Misc:** allergic reactions.	**PO (Adults):** *Psychoses*—2–16 mg 2-4 times daily (not to exceed 64 mg/day). *Nausea/vomiting*—8–16 mg/day in divided doses (not to exceed 24 mg/day). **IM (Adults):** *Psychoses*—5–10 mg initially; may repeat q 6 hr (not to exceed 15–30 mg/day). *Nausea/vomiting*—5 mg initially; may be increased to 10 mg if needed. **IV (Adults):** *Severe nausea/vomiting/hiccups*—1 mg at 1–2-min intervals to a total of 5 mg or as an infusion at a rate not to exceed 1 mg/min (not to exceed 5 mg total dose).

NOTES: **Contraindications:** Hypersensitivity; hypersensitivity to bisulfites (injection); known alcohol intolerance (concentrate only); cross-sensitivity with other phenothiazines may occur; glaucoma; bone marrow depression; severe liver/cardiovascular disease; intestinal obstruction. **Use Cautiously in:** Geriatric, emaciated, or debilitated patients; diabetes; respiratory disease; prostatic hypertrophy; CNS tumors; epilepsy; pregnancy, lactation, or children <12 yr.

Drug	Uses	Side effects	Dosage
plasma protein fraction Plasmanate, Plasma-Plex, Plasmatein, Protenate *Volume expanders* Pregnancy category C	Expansion of plasma volume and maintenance of cardiac output in situations associated with deficiencies in circulatory volume including:	**CNS:** headache. **CV:** hypotension, tachycardia, vascular overload. **GI:** excess salivation, nausea, vomiting. **Derm:** erythema, urticaria. **MS:** back pain. **Misc:** chills, fever, flushing,	Dose is highly individualized depending on condition. Contains 130–160 mEq sodium/liter. Not to exceed 250 g/24 hr. **IV (Adults):** *Hypovolemia*—250–500 ml (12.5–25 g protein). *Hypoproteinemia*—1000–1500 ml (50–75 g pro-

(continued)

{ } available in Canada only. *CAPITALS indicate life-threatening, underlines indicate most frequent

ADDITIONAL DRUGS (CONTINUED)

Generic name Trade name(s) *Classification* Pregnancy category Scheduled substance	Indications	Adverse Reactions and Side Effects[a]	Route and Dosage
plasma protein fraction (continued) Plasmanate, Plasma-Plex, Plasmatein, Protenate *Volume expanders* Pregnancy category C	Shock, hemorrhage, burns Temporary replacement therapy in edema associated with low plasma proteins, such as the nephrotic syndrome and end-stage liver disease.		**IV (Infants and Young Children):** *Hypovolemia*—10–30 ml/kg (0.5–1.5 g protein/kg).

NOTES: Contraindications: Allergic reactions to albumin; normal or increased intravascular volume; CHF; normal or increased intravascular volume; cardiopulmonary bypass procedures. **Cautions:** Severe hepatic/renal disease; rapid infusion; dehydration; large doses.

primidone {Apo-Primidone}, Mysoline, {PMS Primidone}, {Sertan} *Anticonvulsants* Pregnancy category D	Management of tonic-clonic, complex partial, and focal seizures. **Unlabeled Uses:** Management of essential (familial) tremor.	**CNS:** ataxia, drowsiness, vertigo, excitement (increased in children). **EENT:** visual changes. **Resp:** dyspnea. **CV:** edema, orthostatic hypotension. **GI:** anorexia, drug-induced hepatitis, nausea, vomiting. **Derm:** alopecia, rashes. **Hemat:** blood dyscrasias, megaloblastic anemia. **Misc:** folic acid deficiency.	**PO (Adults and Children >8 yr):** Initial dose of 100–125 mg hs for 3 days, then 100–125 mg bid for 3 days, then 100–125 mg tid for 3 days, then maintenance dose of 250 mg 3 times daily (not to exceed 2 g/day). **PO (Children <8 yr):** Initial dose of 50 mg hs for 3 days, then 50 mg bid for next 3 days, then 100 mg bid for 3 days, then maintenance dose of 125–250 mg tid (10–25 mg/kg/day).

NOTES: Contraindications: Hypersensitivity; porphyria. **Use Cautiously in:** Severe liver disease; pregnancy and lactation (may cause hemorrhage in newborn).

probucol Lorelco *Lipid-lowering agents* Pregnancy category B	Adjunct therapy of primary hypercholesterolemia.	**CNS:** dizziness, headache, insomnia. **EENT:** blurred vision, conjunctivitis, decreased sense of smell, lacrimation, tinnitus. **CV:** arrhythmias, ECG changes (prolonged QT interval). **GI:** abdominal pain, bloating, diarrhea, nausea, altered taste, flatulence, GI bleeding, indigestion, vomiting. **Derm:** pruritus, rashes, sweating. **Endo:** enlargement of goiter.	**PO (Adults):** 500 mg twice daily.

Hemat: anemia, eosinophilia, thrombocytopenia.
Neuro: paresthesia, peripheral neuritis.

NOTES: Contraindications: Hypersensitivity; primary biliary cirrhosis; pregnancy; lactation. **Use Cautiously in:** Arrhythmias; untreated congestive heart failure; children.

promazine Primazine, Prozine, Sparine *Antipsychotic agents* *(phenothiazine)* Pregnancy category C	Treatment of various psychotic disorders.	**CNS:** NEUROLEPTIC MALIGNANT SYNDROME, confusion, disorientation, sedation, dizziness, extrapyramidal reactions, fatigue, insomnia, nervousness. **EENT:** blurred vision, diplopia, tinnitus. **CV:** bradycardia, hypertension, hypotension, tachycardia. **GI:** constipation, drug-induced hepatitis, dry mouth. **Derm:** photosensitivity, rashes. **Hemat:** blood dyscrasias.	**PO, IM (Adults):** 10–200 mg q 4–6 hr. **PO, IM (Children > 12 yr):** 10–25 mg q 4–6 hr.

NOTES: Contraindications: Hypersensitivity; cross-sensitivity with other phenothiazines may occur; glaucoma; bone marrow depression; severe liver or cardiovascular disease. **Cautions:** Geriatric/emaciated/debilitated patients; diabetes; respiratory disease; prostatic hypertrophy; CNS tumors; epilepsy; intestinal obstruction; pregnancy or lactation.

propiomazine Largon *Anti-anxiety and sedative/hypnotic* *agent (phenothiazine)* Pregnancy category UK	Used as a sedative preoperatively or during surgery (with opioid analgesics). As an adjunct to analgesics in the management of labor.	**CNS:** NEUROLEPTIC MALIGNANT SYNDROME, drowsiness. **CV:** hypertension, tachycardia. **GI:** dry mouth.	**IM, IV (Adults):** *Preoperative sedation*—20–40 mg. *Sedation during surgery*—10–20 mg. *Obstetric analgesia adjunct*—20–40 mg; may be repeated q 3 hr. **IM, IV (Children):** *Preoperative, preanesthetic, postoperative sedation*—0.55–1.1 mg/kg.

NOTES: Contraindications: Hypersensitivity; cross-sensitivity with other phenothiazines may occur. **Cautions:** Underlying CNS depression; first trimester of pregnancy.

selegiline [Apo-Selegiline], Carbex, Eldepryl, [Gen-Selegiline], [Nu-Selegiline], [Novo-Selegiline], [SD-Deprenyl] *Antiparkinson agents (monoamine oxidase type B inhibitors)* Pregnancy category C	Management of Parkinson's disease (with levodopa or levodopa/carbidopa) in patients who fail to respond to levodopa/carbidopa alone.	**CNS:** confusion, dizziness, fainting, hallucinations, insomnia, vivid dreams. **GI:** nausea, abdominal pain, dry mouth.	**PO (Adults):** 5 mg bid, with breakfast and lunch (some patients may require further dividing of doses 2.5 mg 4 times daily).

NOTES: Contraindications: Hypersensitivity; concurrent opioid therapy; concurrent use of SSRI/tricyclic antidepressants. **Cautions:** Doses >10 mg/day; ulcer disease

sodium fluoride (oral) [Fluor-A-Day], Fluoride Loz, Fluoritab, Flura, Flura-Drops, Flura-Loz, Karidium, Luride, Pediaflor, Pedi-Dent, Pharmaflur, Phos-Flur, [Solu-Flur] *Dental caries prophylactic agents* *Mineral supplements* Pregnancy category UK	Prevention of dental caries in children where insufficient fluoride is available in drinking water.	**CNS:** headache, weakness. **GI:** gastric distress. **Derm:** atopic dermatitis, eczema, urticaria. **Misc:** mottling of teeth (toxicity).	*Fluoride Content of Drinking Water: <0.3 ppm* **PO (Adults and Children >16 yr):** No supplementation. **PO (Children 6–16 yr):** 1 mg/day. **PO (Children 3–6 yr):** 0.5 mg/day. **PO (Children 6 mo–3 yr):** 0.25 mg/day. **PO (Children <6 mo):** No supplementation.

{} available in Canada only. *CAPITALS indicate life-threatening, underlines indicate most frequent

(continued)

ADDITIONAL DRUGS (CONTINUED)

Generic name Trade name(s) Classification Pregnancy category Scheduled substance	Indications	Adverse Reactions and Side Effects*	Route and Dosage
sodium fluoride (oral) (continued) [Fluor-A-Day], Fluoride Loz, Fluori-tab, Flura, Flura-Drops, Flura-Loz, Karidium, Luride, Pediaflor, Pedi-Dent, Pharmaflur, Phos-Flur, [Solu-Flur] *Dental caries prophylactic agents* *Mineral supplements* Pregnancy category UK			***Fluoride Content of Drinking Water: 0.3–0.6 ppm*** **PO (Adults and Children >16 yr):** No supplementation. **PO (Children 6–16 yr):** 0.5 mg/day. **PO (Children 3–6 yr):** 0.25 mg/day. **PO (Children <3 yr):** No supplementation.

NOTES: Contraindications: Hypersensitivity; dietary sodium restriction; where fluoride in drinking water exceeds 0.7 parts per million; some products contain tartrazine and should be avoided in patients with known intolerance; severe renal impairment. **Cautions:** Situations where fluoride content of water is unknown.

spectinomycin Trobicin *Anti-infective agents* Pregnancy category B	Second-line treatment of gonorrhea and gonococcal urethritis, cervicitis, or proctitis in patients who are infected with penicillin-resistant strains of *Neisseria gonorrhoeae.* Treatment of gonorrhea and gonococcal urethritis, cervicitis, or proctitis in patients allergic to beta-lactam anti-infectives (including ceftriaxone).	**CNS:** dizziness, headache, insomnia, nervousness. **GI:** nausea, vomiting. **Derm:** pruritus, transient rashes, urticaria. **Local:** pain at IM site. **Misc:** hypersensitivity reactions, including ANAPHY-LAXIS, chills, fever.	**IM (Adults and Children >45 kg):** 2-g single dose (2 g q 12 hr for 3 days for disseminated gonorrhea). **IM (Infants and Children <45 kg):** 40 mg/kg single dose.

NOTES: Contraindications: Hypersensitivity; neonates (diluent contains benzyl alcohol). **Cautions:** Concurrent infection with other sexually transmitted disease (additional anti-infectives required); pregnancy, lactation, or children (has been used safely).

triprolidine *Antihistamines* Pregnancy category B	Symptomatic relief of allergic symptoms caused by histamine release Most useful in management of nasal allergies and allergic dermatoses. Available only in combination with other agents (decongestants).	**CNS:** drowsiness, dizziness, excitation (↑ in children). **EENT:** blurred vision. **CV:** arrhythmias, hypertension, hypotension, palpitations. **GI:** dry mouth, constipation.	**PO (Adults):** 2.5 mg q 4-6 hr (not to exceed 10 mg/24 hr). **PO (Children 6–12 yr):** 1.25 mg q 6–8 hr (not to exceed 5 mg/24 hr). **PO (Children 4–6 yr):** 937 mcg q 6–8 hr (not to exceed 3.75 mg/24 hr).

| | GU: hesitancy, retention. | PO (Children 2–4 yr): 625 mcg q 6–8 hr (not to exceed 2.5 mg/24 hr).
PO (Children 4 mo–2 yr): 312 mcg q 6–8 hr (not to exceed 1.25 mg/24 hr.) |

NOTES: Contraindications: Hypersensitivity; acute asthma; lactation; known alcohol intolerance (some liquids). **Cautions:** Geriatric patients; glaucoma; liver disease; prostatic hypertrophy.

| valrubicin
Valstar
Antineoplastic agents (antbracycline)
Pregnancy category C | Intravesicular (bladder instillation) therapy of bacille Calmette-Guérin (BCG)-refractory carcinoma in situ of the urinary bladder in patients for whom surgery is inappropriate. | Intravesicular (Adults): 800 mg instilled into urinary bladder once weekly for 6 wk. | CNS: dizziness, headache, malaise, weakness.
Resp: pneumonia.
CV: chest pain, vasodilation.
GI: abdominal pain, diarrhea, flatulence, nausea, vomiting.
GU: bladder spasm, cystitis, dysuria, hematuria, red urine, urinary incontinence, urinary tract infection, urinary urgency, local burning, nocturia, urethral pain, urinary retention.
Derm: rash.
F and E: peripheral edema.
Hemat: anemia.
Metab: hyperglycemia.
MS: back pain. |

NOTES: Contraindications: Hypersensitivity to anthracyclines or Cremophor EL; known alcohol intolerance; concurrent urinary tract infection; perforated bladder/conditions where the integrity of the bladder mucosa has been compromised; pregnancy and lactation; recent transurethral resection and/or fulguration. **Cautions:** Patients with severe irritable bladder symptoms; childbearing potential, children.

| vitamin A
Aquasol A
Vitamins (fat soluble)
Pregnancy category A (oral), X (parenteral, or doses > RDA) | Treatment and prevention of deficiency states. Prevention of vitamin A deficiency in patients who have fat malabsorption or are taking bile acid sequestrants. | Misc: hypervitaminosis A syndrome. | RE = retinol equivalents.
PO (Adults): *Deficiency*—If xerophthalmia is present, 7500–15,000 RE (25,000–50,000 units/day).
PO (Children 1 yr): *Measles*—60,000 RE (200,000 units) single dose. *Xerophthalmia*—60,000 RE (200,000 units) daily for 2 days; repeat at 4 wk.
PO (Children 6 mo–1 yr): *Measles*—30,000 RE (100,000 units) single dose. *Xerophthalmia* 30,000 RE (100,000 units) daily for 2 days; repeat at 4 wk.
IM (Adults and Children 8 yr): 15,000–30,000 RE (50,000–100,000 units)/day for 3 days; then 15,000 RE (50,000 units)/day for 2 wk.
IM (Children 1–8 yr): 5000–35,000 units/day for 10 days. |

(continued)

() available in Canada only. *CAPITALS indicate life-threatening, underlines indicate most frequent

ADDITIONAL DRUGS (CONTINUED)

Generic name Trade name(s) Classification Pregnancy category Scheduled substance	Indications	Adverse Reactions and Side Effects*	Route and Dosage
vitamin A (continued) Aquasol A Vitamins (fat soluble) Pregnancy category A (oral), X (parenteral, or doses > RDA)			IM (Children <1 yr): 1500–4500 RE (5000–15,000 units)/ day for 10 days. IV (Adults and Children): Infused as part of TPN in amounts required to meet nutritional needs (in parenteral multivita- min preparations).

NOTES: Contraindications: Hypervitaminosis A; malabsorption (oral products); hypersensitivity to ingredients in preparations. Cautions: Lactation; pregnancy; severely impaired renal function. Doses should be individualized on the basis of deficiency.

zileuton Zyflo Bronchodilators (enzyme inhibitor) Pregnancy category C	Long-term control agent in the management of asthma.	CNS: headache, dizziness, insomnia, malaise, nerv- ousness, somnolence. EENT: conjunctivitis. CV: chest pain. GI: abdominal pain, constipation, dyspepsia, flatu- lence, increased liver enzymes, nausea, vomiting. GU: urinary tract infection, vaginitis. Derm: pruritus. MS: arthralgia, myalgia, neck pain. Neuro: hypertonia. Misc: fever, lymphadenopathy.	PO (Adults and Children ≥12 yr): 600 mg 4 times daily.

NOTES: Contraindications: Hypersensitivity, liver disease. Cautions: Acute asthma, history of liver disease/ alcohol consumption; pregnancy, lactation, or children <12 yr.

{ } available in Canada only. *CAPITALS indicate life-threatening, underlines indicate most frequent

COMPREHENSIVE INDEX*

generic / Trade / *classification*

---

*Entries for **generic** names appear in **boldface type**, trade names appear in regular type, CLASSIFICATIONS appear in BOLDFACE SMALL CAPS, Combination Drugs appear in *italics*, and herbal products are preceded by a leaf icon (✤). A "C" and a **boldface** page number following a generic name identify the page in the "Classification" section on which that drug is listed.

---

*Entries for **generic** names appear in **boldface type**, trade names appear in regular type, CLASSIFICATIONS appear in BOLDFACE SMALL CAPS, Combination Drugs appear in *italics,* and herbal products are preceded by a leaf icon (❧). A "C" and a **boldface** page number following a generic name identify the page in the "Classification" section on which that drug is listed.

---

*Entries for **generic** names appear in **boldface type**, trade names appear in regular type, CLASSIFICATIONS appear in **BOLDFACE SMALL CAPS**, Combination Drugs appear in *italics*, and herbal products are preceded by a leaf icon (✤). A "C" and a **boldface** page number following a generic name identify the page in the "Classification" section on which that drug is listed.

---

*Entries for **generic** names appear in **boldface type**, trade names appear in regular type, CLASSIFICATIONS appear in BOLDFACE SMALL CAPS, Combination Drugs appear in *italics,* and herbal products are preceded by a leaf icon (✤). A "C" and a **boldface** page number following a generic name identify the page in the "Classification" section on which that drug is listed.

*Entries for **generic** names appear in **boldface type,** trade names appear in regular type, CLASSIFICATIONS appear in **BOLDFACE SMALL CAPS,** Combination Drugs appear in *italics,* and herbal products are preceded by a leaf icon (♣). A "C" and a **boldface** page number following a generic name identify the page in the "Classification" section on which that drug is listed.

---

*Entries for **generic** names appear in **boldface type**, trade names appear in regular type, CLASSIFICATIONS appear in BOLDFACE SMALL CAPS, Combination Drugs appear in *italics*, and herbal products are preceded by a leaf icon (✤). A "C" and a **boldface** page number following a generic name identify the page in the "Classification" section on which that drug is listed.

---

*Entries for **generic** names appear in **boldface type,** trade names appear in regular type, CLASSIFICATIONS appear in BOLDFACE SMALL CAPS, Combination Drugs appear in *italics,* and herbal products are preceded by a leaf icon (❧). A "**C**" and a **boldface** page number following a generic name identify the page in the "Classification" section on which that drug is listed.

---

*Entries for **generic** names appear in **boldface type,** trade names appear in regular type, CLASSIFICATIONS appear in BOLDFACE SMALL CAPS, Combination Drugs appear in *italics,* and herbal products are preceded by a leaf icon (✤). A "C" and a **boldface** page number following a generic name identify the page in the "Classification" section on which that drug is listed.

---

*Entries for **generic** names appear in **boldface type,** trade names appear in regular type, CLASSIFICATIONS appear in BOLDFACE SMALL CAPS, Combination Drugs appear in *italics,* and herbal products are preceded by a leaf icon (✦). A "C" and a **boldface** page number following a generic name identify the page in the "Classification" section on which that drug is listed.

---

*Entries for **generic** names appear in **boldface type,** trade names appear in regular type, CLASSIFICATIONS appear in BOLDFACE SMALL CAPS, Combination Drugs appear in *italics,* and herbal products are preceded by a leaf icon (✤). A "C" and a **boldface** page number following a generic name identify the page in the "Classification" section on which that drug is listed.

---

*Entries for **generic** names appear in **boldface type,** trade names appear in regular type,
CLASSIFICATIONS appear in BOLDFACE SMALL CAPS, Combination Drugs appear in *italics,* and herbal
products are preceded by a leaf icon (♣). A "C" and a **boldface** page number following a generic
name identify the page in the "Classification" section on which that drug is listed.

*Entries for **generic** names appear in **boldface type,** trade names appear in regular type, CLASSIFICATIONS appear in BOLDFACE SMALL CAPS, Combination Drugs appear in *italics,* and herbal products are preceded by a leaf icon (♣). A "C" and a **boldface** page number following a generic name identify the page in the "Classification" section on which that drug is listed.

---

*Entries for **generic** names appear in **boldface type**, trade names appear in regular type, CLASSIFICATIONS appear in BOLDFACE SMALL CAPS, Combination Drugs appear in *italics*, and herbal products are preceded by a leaf icon (♣). A "C" and a **boldface** page number following a generic name identify the page in the "Classification" section on which that drug is listed.

---

*Entries for **generic** names appear in **boldface type**, trade names appear in regular type, CLASSIFICATIONS appear in BOLDFACE SMALL CAPS, Combination Drugs appear in *italics*, and herbal products are preceded by a leaf icon (♣). A "C" and a **boldface** page number following a generic name identify the page in the "Classification" section on which that drug is listed.

---

*Entries for **generic** names appear in **boldface type,** trade names appear in regular type, **CLASSIFICATIONS** appear in **BOLDFACE SMALL CAPS,** Combination Drugs appear in *italics,* and herbal products are preceded by a leaf icon (✤). A "**C**" and a **boldface** page number following a generic name identify the page in the "Classification" section on which that drug is listed.

*Entries for **generic** names appear in **boldface type,** trade names appear in regular type, CLASSIFICATIONS appear in BOLDFACE SMALL CAPS, Combination Drugs appear in *italics,* and herbal products are preceded by a leaf icon (🍃). A "C" and a **boldface** page number following a generic name identify the page in the "Classification" section on which that drug is listed.

---

*Entries for **generic** names appear in **boldface type,** trade names appear in regular type, **CLASSIFICATIONS** appear in **BOLDFACE SMALL CAPS,** Combination Drugs appear in *italics,* and herbal products are preceded by a leaf icon (✤). A "C" and a **boldface** page number following a generic name identify the page in the "Classification" section on which that drug is listed.

---

*Entries for **generic** names appear in **boldface type,** trade names appear in regular type, CLASSIFICATIONS appear in **BOLDFACE SMALL CAPS**, Combination Drugs appear in *italics,* and herbal products are preceded by a leaf icon (❧). A "C" and a **boldface** page number following a generic name identify the page in the "Classification" section on which that drug is listed.

---

*Entries for **generic** names appear in **boldface type,** trade names appear in regular type, CLASSIFICATIONS appear in BOLDFACE SMALL CAPS, Combination Drugs appear in *italics,* and herbal products are preceded by a leaf icon (♣). A "C" and a **boldface** page number following a generic name identify the page in the "Classification" section on which that drug is listed.

*Entries for **generic** names appear in **boldface type**, trade names appear in regular type,
CLASSIFICATIONS appear in **BOLDFACE SMALL CAPS**, Combination Drugs appear in *italics,* and herbal
products are preceded by a leaf icon (✤). A "C" and a **boldface** page number following a generic
name identify the page in the "Classification" section on which that drug is listed.

---

*Entries for **generic** names appear in **boldface type,** trade names appear in regular type, CLASSIFICATIONS appear in BOLDFACE SMALL CAPS, Combination Drugs appear in *italics,* and herbal products are preceded by a leaf icon (♣). A "C" and a **boldface** page number following a generic name identify the page in the "Classification" section on which that drug is listed.

---

*Entries for **generic** names appear in **boldface type**, trade names appear in regular type, CLASSIFICATIONS appear in BOLDFACE SMALL CAPS, Combination Drugs appear in *italics*, and herbal products are preceded by a leaf icon (♣). A "C" and a **boldface** page number following a generic name identify the page in the "Classification" section on which that drug is listed.

---

*Entries for **generic** names appear in **boldface type**, trade names appear in regular type,
CLASSIFICATIONS appear in BOLDFACE SMALL CAPS, Combination Drugs appear in *italics,* and herbal
products are preceded by a leaf icon (✤). A "C" and a **boldface** page number following a generic
name identify the page in the "Classification" section on which that drug is listed.

---

*Entries for **generic** names appear in **boldface type**, trade names appear in regular type, CLASSIFICATIONS appear in **BOLDFACE SMALL CAPS**, Combination Drugs appear in *italics*, and herbal products are preceded by a leaf icon (✤). A "C" and a **boldface** page number following a generic name identify the page in the "Classification" section on which that drug is listed.

*Entries for **generic** names appear in **boldface type**, trade names appear in regular type,
CLASSIFICATIONS appear in **BOLDFACE SMALL CAPS**, Combination Drugs appear in *italics*, and herbal
products are preceded by a leaf icon (✤). A "C" and a **boldface** page number following a generic
name identify the page in the "Classification" section on which that drug is listed.

---

*Entries for **generic** names appear in **boldface type**, trade names appear in regular type, CLASSIFICATIONS appear in **BOLDFACE SMALL CAPS**, Combination Drugs appear in *italics,* and herbal products are preceded by a leaf icon (✤). A "C" and a **boldface** page number following a generic name identify the page in the "Classification" section on which that drug is listed.

---

*Entries for **generic** names appear in **boldface type,** trade names appear in regular type, CLASSIFICATIONS appear in **BOLDFACE SMALL CAPS**, Combination Drugs appear in *italics,* and herbal products are preceded by a leaf icon (✤). A "C" and a **boldface** page number following a generic name identify the page in the "Classification" section on which that drug is listed.

---

*Entries for **generic** names appear in **boldface type**, trade names appear in regular type, CLASSIFICATIONS appear in BOLDFACE SMALL CAPS, Combination Drugs appear in *italics*, and herbal products are preceded by a leaf icon (✤). A "C" and a **boldface** page number following a generic name identify the page in the "Classification" section on which that drug is listed.

---

*Entries for **generic** names appear in **boldface type**, trade names appear in regular type, CLASSIFICATIONS appear in BOLDFACE SMALL CAPS, Combination Drugs appear in *italics*, and herbal products are preceded by a leaf icon (♣). A "C" and a **boldface** page number following a generic name identify the page in the "Classification" section on which that drug is listed.

---

*Entries for **generic** names appear in **boldface type**, trade names appear in regular type, CLASSIFICATIONS appear in BOLDFACE SMALL CAPS, Combination Drugs appear in *italics,* and herbal products are preceded by a leaf icon (❧). A "C" and a **boldface** page number following a generic name identify the page in the "Classification" section on which that drug is listed.

*Entries for **generic** names appear in **boldface type,** trade names appear in regular type, CLASSIFICATIONS appear in BOLDFACE SMALL CAPS, Combination Drugs appear in *italics,* and herbal products are preceded by a leaf icon (♣). A "C" and a **boldface** page number following a generic name identify the page in the "Classification" section on which that drug is listed.

---

*Entries for **generic** names appear in **boldface type,** trade names appear in regular type, CLASSIFICATIONS appear in BOLDFACE SMALL CAPS, Combination Drugs appear in *italics,* and herbal products are preceded by a leaf icon (✤). A "C" and a **boldface** page number following a generic name identify the page in the "Classification" section on which that drug is listed.

*Entries for **generic** names appear in **boldface type**, trade names appear in regular type, CLASSIFICATIONS appear in BOLDFACE SMALL CAPS, Combination Drugs appear in *italics,* and herbal products are preceded by a leaf icon (✤). A "C" and a **boldface** page number following a generic name identify the page in the "Classification" section on which that drug is listed.

*Entries for **generic** names appear in **boldface type**, trade names appear in regular type, CLASSIFICATIONS appear in BOLDFACE SMALL CAPS, Combination Drugs appear in *italics*, and herbal products are preceded by a leaf icon (✤). A "C" and a **boldface** page number following a generic name identify the page in the "Classification" section on which that drug is listed.

---

*Entries for **generic** names appear in **boldface type**, trade names appear in regular type, CLASSIFICATIONS appear in **BOLDFACE SMALL CAPS**, Combination Drugs appear in *italics*, and herbal products are preceded by a leaf icon (✿). A "**C**" and a **boldface** page number following a generic name identify the page in the "Classification" section on which that drug is listed.

---

*Entries for **generic** names appear in **boldface type**, trade names appear in regular type, CLASSIFICATIONS appear in BOLDFACE SMALL CAPS, Combination Drugs appear in *italics*, and herbal products are preceded by a leaf icon (✤). A "C" and a **boldface** page number following a generic name identify the page in the "Classification" section on which that drug is listed.

*Entries for **generic** names appear in **boldface type,** trade names appear in regular type, CLASSIFICATIONS appear in **BOLDFACE SMALL CAPS,** Combination Drugs appear in *italics,* and herbal products are preceded by a leaf icon (✤). A "C" and a **boldface** page number following a generic name identify the page in the "Classification" section on which that drug is listed.

---

*Entries for **generic** names appear in **boldface type**, trade names appear in regular type, CLASSIFICATIONS appear in **BOLDFACE SMALL CAPS**, Combination Drugs appear in *italics,* and herbal products are preceded by a leaf icon (✤). A "C" and a **boldface** page number following a generic name identify the page in the "Classification" section on which that drug is listed.

*Entries for **generic** names appear in **boldface type,** trade names appear in regular type, CLASSIFICATIONS appear in BOLDFACE SMALL CAPS, Combination Drugs appear in *italics,* and herbal products are preceded by a leaf icon (♣). A "C" and a **boldface** page number following a generic name identify the page in the "Classification" section on which that drug is listed.

---

*Entries for **generic** names appear in **boldface type,** trade names appear in regular type, CLASSIFICATIONS appear in BOLDFACE SMALL CAPS, Combination Drugs appear in *italics,* and herbal products are preceded by a leaf icon (❦). A "C" and a **boldface** page number following a generic name identify the page in the "Classification" section on which that drug is listed.

---

*Entries for **generic** names appear in **boldface type,** trade names appear in regular type, CLASSIFICATIONS appear in BOLDFACE SMALL CAPS, Combination Drugs appear in *italics,* and herbal products are preceded by a leaf icon (✤). A "C" and a **boldface** page number following a generic name identify the page in the "Classification" section on which that drug is listed.

---

*Entries for **generic** names appear in **boldface type,** trade names appear in regular type,
CLASSIFICATIONS appear in **BOLDFACE SMALL CAPS**, Combination Drugs appear in *italics*, and herbal
products are preceded by a leaf icon (♣). A "**C**" and a **boldface** page number following a generic
name identify the page in the "Classification" section on which that drug is listed.

---

*Entries for **generic** names appear in **boldface type**, trade names appear in regular type, CLASSIFICATIONS appear in BOLDFACE SMALL CAPS, Combination Drugs appear in *italics*, and herbal products are preceded by a leaf icon (♣). A "C" and a **boldface** page number following a generic name identify the page in the "Classification" section on which that drug is listed.

---

*Entries for **generic** names appear in **boldface type,** trade names appear in regular type, CLASSIFICATIONS appear in BOLDFACE SMALL CAPS, Combination Drugs appear in *italics,* and herbal products are preceded by a leaf icon (🍁). A "C" and a **boldface** page number following a generic name identify the page in the "Classification" section on which that drug is listed.

---

*Entries for **generic** names appear in **boldface type,** trade names appear in regular type,
CLASSIFICATIONS appear in BOLDFACE SMALL CAPS, Combination Drugs appear in *italics,* and herbal
products are preceded by a leaf icon (✤). A "C" and a **boldface** page number following a generic
name identify the page in the "Classification" section on which that drug is listed.

*Entries for **generic** names appear in **boldface type,** trade names appear in regular type, CLASSIFICATIONS appear in BOLDFACE SMALL CAPS, Combination Drugs appear in *italics,* and herbal products are preceded by a leaf icon (♣). A "C" and a **boldface** page number following a generic name identify the page in the "Classification" section on which that drug is listed.

---

*Entries for **generic** names appear in **boldface type,** trade names appear in regular type,
CLASSIFICATIONS appear in BOLDFACE SMALL CAPS, Combination Drugs appear in *italics,* and herbal
products are preceded by a leaf icon (♣). A "C" and a **boldface** page number following a generic
name identify the page in the "Classification" section on which that drug is listed.

*Entries for **generic** names appear in **boldface type**, trade names appear in regular type,
CLASSIFICATIONS appear in BOLDFACE SMALL CAPS, Combination Drugs appear in *italics,* and herbal
products are preceded by a leaf icon (✤). A "C" and a **boldface** page number following a generic
name identify the page in the "Classification" section on which that drug is listed.

---

*Entries for **generic** names appear in **boldface type**, trade names appear in regular type, CLASSIFICATIONS appear in **BOLDFACE SMALL CAPS**, Combination Drugs appear in *italics*, and herbal products are preceded by a leaf icon (✤). A "C" and a **boldface** page number following a generic name identify the page in the "Classification" section on which that drug is listed.

---

*Entries for **generic** names appear in **boldface type**, trade names appear in regular type, CLASSIFICATIONS appear in BOLDFACE SMALL CAPS, Combination Drugs appear in *italics*, and herbal products are preceded by a leaf icon (✤). A "C" and a **boldface** page number following a generic name identify the page in the "Classification" section on which that drug is listed.

---

*Entries for **generic** names appear in **boldface type**, trade names appear in regular type, CLASSIFICATIONS appear in BOLDFACE SMALL CAPS, Combination Drugs appear in *italics,* and herbal products are preceded by a leaf icon (✤). A "C" and a **boldface** page number following a generic name identify the page in the "Classification" section on which that drug is listed.

---

*Entries for **generic** names appear in **boldface type,** trade names appear in regular type, CLASSIFICATIONS appear in **BOLDFACE SMALL CAPS**, Combination Drugs appear in *italics,* and herbal products are preceded by a leaf icon (✤). A "C" and a **boldface** page number following a generic name identify the page in the "Classification" section on which that drug is listed.

---

*Entries for **generic** names appear in **boldface type,** trade names appear in regular type, CLASSIFICATIONS appear in **BOLDFACE SMALL CAPS,** Combination Drugs appear in *italics,* and herbal products are preceded by a leaf icon (❧). A "C" and a **boldface** page number following a generic name identify the page in the "Classification" section on which that drug is listed.

---

*Entries for **generic** names appear in **boldface type**, trade names appear in regular type, CLASSIFICATIONS appear in BOLDFACE SMALL CAPS, Combination Drugs appear in *italics*, and herbal products are preceded by a leaf icon (❀). A "**C**" and a boldface page number following a generic name identify the page in the "Classification" section on which that drug is listed.

---

*Entries for **generic** names appear in **boldface type,** trade names appear in regular type, CLASSIFICATIONS appear in BOLDFACE SMALL CAPS, Combination Drugs appear in *italics,* and herbal products are preceded by a leaf icon (❧). A "C" and a **boldface** page number following a generic name identify the page in the "Classification" section on which that drug is listed.

*Entries for **generic** names appear in **boldface type,** trade names appear in regular type, CLASSIFICATIONS appear in BOLDFACE SMALL CAPS, Combination Drugs appear in *italics,* and herbal products are preceded by a leaf icon (♣). A "C" and a **boldface** page number following a generic name identify the page in the "Classification" section on which that drug is listed.

*Entries for **generic** names appear in **boldface type,** trade names appear in regular type, CLASSIFICATIONS appear in **BOLDFACE SMALL CAPS,** Combination Drugs appear in *italics,* and herbal products are preceded by a leaf icon (✤). A "C" and a **boldface** page number following a generic name identify the page in the "Classification" section on which that drug is listed.

*Entries for **generic** names appear in **boldface type**, trade names appear in regular type, CLASSIFICATIONS appear in BOLDFACE SMALL CAPS, Combination Drugs appear in *italics,* and herbal products are preceded by a leaf icon (♣). A "C" and a **boldface** page number following a generic name identify the page in the "Classification" section on which that drug is listed.

---

*Entries for **generic** names appear in **boldface type,** trade names appear in regular type, CLASSIFICATIONS appear in BOLDFACE SMALL CAPS, Combination Drugs appear in *italics,* and herbal products are preceded by a leaf icon (✤). A "C" and a **boldface** page number following a generic name identify the page in the "Classification" section on which that drug is listed.

*Entries for **generic** names appear in **boldface type**, trade names appear in regular type, CLASSIFICATIONS appear in BOLDFACE SMALL CAPS, Combination Drugs appear in *italics*, and herbal products are preceded by a leaf icon (♣). A "C" and a **boldface** page number following a generic name identify the page in the "Classification" section on which that drug is listed.

*Entries for **generic** names appear in **boldface type,** trade names appear in regular type, CLASSIFICATIONS appear in BOLDFACE SMALL CAPS, Combination Drugs appear in *italics,* and herbal products are preceded by a leaf icon (✤). A "**C**" and a **boldface** page number following a generic name identify the page in the "Classification" section on which that drug is listed.

NOTES

NOTES